The FOOT DOCTOR

Lifetime Relief for Your Aching Feet

by
Dr. Glenn Copeland, D.P.M.
with
Stan Solomon

Illustrations by Lori McKay

 Rodale Press, Emmaus, Pennsylvania

Library of Congress Cataloging-in-Publication Data

Copeland, Glenn.
  The foot doctor.

  Includes index.
  1. Foot—Care and hygiene. 2. Foot—Diseases.
I. Solomon, Stan. II. Title.
RD563.C67 1986   617′.585   86-6461
ISBN 0-87857-663-0 paperback

Design: Don Fernley

Printed in Canada

2 4 6 8 10 9 7 5 3 1 paperback

To my parents, Margaret and Lou,
my wife, Ruthie,
my children, Elyssa, Lauren, and Aaron,
and to the memory of my eldest brother,
E. Vernon Copeland,
who will be a part of me always.

Contents

Foreword by Dr. Hamilton Hall

I met Glenn Copeland when he joined the staff at Women's College Hospital in Toronto. From the beginning, Glenn was enthusiastic to educate the public, including the medical profession, about the role of podiatry and its approach to foot problems. As an orthopedic surgeon, I constantly hear complaints about sore feet, so I was intrigued with Glenn's approach and impressed with his fresh ideas.

The result of our early collaboration was a Lower Limb Clinic which opened at Women's College Hospital in 1977. I witnessed Glenn's thorough knowledge of the biomechanical relationship between the foot and function in the knees, hips, and low back. While I didn't always agree with his approach, I couldn't argue with his success. I still recall one of our original patients who arrived in the clinic with both sore feet and low-back pain. Glenn noticed that the patient's feet pronated excessively whenever she walked and suggested a particular type of running-shoe to correct the problem. He also predicted that this correction would relieve her back complaints. Although I was skeptical, the patient and I agreed to try this simple approach. Six weeks later, her back pain had almost completely disappeared. Of course, this one case didn't prove an exclusive relationship between low-back disorders and biomechanical foot problems, but it did suggest an area of research that Glenn and I have continued to pursue through the Canadian Back Institute, where Glenn is the podiatric consultant.

Over the years, Dr. Copeland and I have had our share of disagreements and have retained our different approaches to the treatment of lower-limb problems. My experience as an orthopedic surgeon sometimes conflicts with Glenn's training as a foot doctor. Our diagnostic and surgical procedures can be quite different, but despite these differences, I value Glenn's judgement and expertise. As a podiatrist, he emphasizes ambulatory outpatient surgery. Only recently have orthopedic surgeons come to recognize the efficiency and cost-effectiveness of these techniques. Dr. Copeland's experience with this approach has heightened his ability to rapidly diagnose and treat common foot ailments. His skill is particularly appreciated in our many sports medicine clinics.

In *The Foot Doctor*, Glenn dispels many myths concerning the feet. He brings a proper perspective to common foot disorders that for years have been misunderstood or mis-diagnosed. If you suffer from foot complaints or leg problems that might be associated with poorly functioning feet, this book may hold the answer. Everyone will find it interesting and very readable, with the information presented in an understandable, entertaining fashion. Sooner or later, most of us will develop foot problems, problems which may be avoided or easily treated with the understanding gained from *The Foot Doctor*.

HAMILTON HALL, M.D., F.R.C.S. (C)
author of *The Back Doctor*

Preface

I had been contemplating a book about foot care for a couple of years when a particular incident occurred in my office which convinced me that the time had come to get serious about putting my thoughts into writing.

In the presence of a young intern who had been assigned to me as a student, I was examining an older female patient for a series of foot complaints, and was taking great pains to explain to her exactly why she was experiencing acute discomfort and what could be done to provide her with relief. At an opportune moment the intern quietly asked me why I was being so explicit with the patient. "Why can't you just tell her she has arthritis and give her some anti-inflammatory pills?" he asked.

After the patient had left, I took the intern aside and explained to him that fear and anxiety of the unknown often bother the patient as much as, if not more than, the actual pain. The patient has a right to know what the problem is, how it can be treated, and that most foot problems can be corrected with conservative measures. But, even if he or she does need surgery, modern surgical techniques rarely require in-patient hospital treatment and lengthy immobile periods of recuperation.

As I listened to myself speaking to the intern, it became clear to me that I had to write this book, because I feel so strongly about the public's need to know enough about their feet to prevent needless misery, and I want to save them from suffering anxiety attacks because of fear of the unknown. The problem they have is most likely common and easily treatable. If, in the process, I manage to educate some medical professionals about foot disorders they have not been trained to deal with adequately, and encourage them to speak frankly with their patients, in easily understandable language, so much the better.

It was a striking coincidence that shortly after my discussion with the intern, I was interviewed for an article exploring the relationship between foot and back problems. The interviewer eventually became my co-author, and *The Foot Doctor* was born.

As you can imagine, I could not have written this book without the knowledge, tutelage, encouragement, and friendship of many people over the years. I would like to single out a few of them to whom I owe a special debt of gratitude.

Ricky Kanee Schachter, M.D., F.R.C.P., the former head of the Dermatology Department at Women's College Hospital in Toronto, first supported my application to join the staff of that hospital. David Moorsom, M.D., F.R.C.P. (Department of Internal Medicine, Women's College Hospital), Jay Taradash, M.D., F.R.C.P. (Department of Dermatology, Women's College Hospital), and Michael Kliman, M.D., F.R.C.S. (Department of Orthopedic Surgery, St. Joseph's Hospital, Toronto), have all contributed ideas for the manuscript, and have been wonderful friends. Morris Zoladek, D.P.M., podiatrist, has also been a great help as an advisor and friend. Moreover, he had the good sense to choose me for a brother-in-law. Ron Taylor, M.D., Family Practitioner, and Allan Gross, M.D., F.R.C.S. (Professor of Orthopedic Surgery, University of Toronto), gave me the opportunity to work with them for the past five years at the S. C. Cooper Family Sports Medicine Clinic at Mount Sinai Hospital in Toronto. I owe a lot of my sports-medicine knowledge to them.

Words cannot adequately express my great appreciation and gratitude to Carol-Ann Reed, M.D., F.R.C.S. (C), and Hamilton Hall, M.D., F.R.C.S. (C), orthopedic surgeon and the author of *The Back Doctor*. No two medical professionals have given me more support, understanding, and encouragement since I have been in practice. They have been like a sister and a brother to me, and their combined efforts on my behalf will never be forgotten.

I would be remiss if I did not thank Kevin Honsberger, physiotherapist, and Peter Charbonneau, athletic therapist, for their help with Chapters Fourteen and Fifteen. Also, working with medical illustrator Lori McKay was fascinating. She had a marvellous grasp of the complexities involved in showing various parts of the foot and what can go wrong with them. Thanks also to my editor and friend at Macmillan, Pat Kennedy, whom I've learned to deeply appreciate for her understanding and support.

As for my co-author, Stan Solomon, his friendship, support, and hundreds of hours of work have made this book a reality. *The Foot Doctor* is as much a part of him as it is of me. I must also thank his wife, Linda, who became a good friend, and who kept him going when his spirits were flagging.

What more can I say about my parents, Margaret and Lou, and my brother Martin than that, without their love, understanding, and support, my achievements in life would have been much more difficult, if not impossible.

Finally, and most importantly, my major sources of inspiration: my childhood sweetheart and wife of twelve years, Ruthie, and my three beautiful kids, Elyssa, Lauren, and Aaron. Where would I be without them? Who could possibly be more understanding of my foibles—and the leisure hours I had to give up to complete this book? I hope we shall now have some time to savor our successes together.

1

Introductory Footnotes

If your feet do not hurt too much, take a stroll through any major bookstore with a large self-help/health-care section. There you will find numerous works devoted to various parts of the body, to the mind, to exercise, to diets, to sex, and/or to combinations thereof. But there is almost nothing on the shelves that focuses specifically on the lowly, unglamorous foot. It is not unusual for the foot to be ignored and abused—many times due to ignorance—because distress in the lower extremities of the body is rarely indicative of critical illness. It is not until acute discomfort forces a person to seek medical attention that he or she becomes aware of what can go wrong with the feet, and how foot problems can be avoided or corrected. Another major factor that contributes to ignorance among the general public is the fact that many medical professionals also lack information about foot problems. They were not required to concentrate on this part of the anatomy in any great detail in medical school, and consequently they devote little attention to the feet of their patients unless severe pain creates major concern. This is not the fault of the medical profession, *per se*. It is quite logical to focus attention on the more serious diseases and dysfunctions that they have found to be common.

So, the general public knows very little about their feet, and this is a sad fact when one considers that about eighty per cent of mankind will suffer from a foot disorder during their lifetimes.

Another sad fact is that when a person has a foot disorder, problems can be created that affect other parts of the body, and even the psyche. We often hear about how much an aching back can affect a person's general well-being. According to most of my patients, the same can be said about feet. I constantly hear the expression "When my feet hurt, I hurt all over" from patients who hobble into my office with various foot problems. In fact, Abe Lincoln is supposed to have said that when his feet hurt he could not think clearly.

Bad feet can impair not only one's thought processes, but one's emotional well-being as well. I examine many athletes with foot problems every week, and most of them are very depressed because they have been forced by an injury to stop running, exercising, or playing their favorite sport. A grounded athlete can turn very quickly into a grouch. I know this from personal experience.

As to other parts of the body being adversely affected by foot disorders, I have found that a foot abnormality can cause problems all the way up to the top of the spinal column, although it is rare to find a relationship between sore feet and a sore neck. It is not uncommon, however, to find a foot abnormality responsible for pain and dysfunction in the legs, knees, hips, and lower back.

Throughout the book I will be discussing the relationship between the feet and other parts of the body, and how a problem in one area of the foot can affect another part of the foot as well. But let me give you a brief example here of how a chain reaction can begin.

A man develops a callus on the bottom of his foot (for reasons that will be discussed in detail in Chapter Seven). Because the area hurts so much, he begins to alter his walking pattern deliberately to avoid putting painful pressure on the callus. As a result, he places undue stress on other parts of the foot, which then also become sore. Now the man alters his gait even further to avoid discomfort when he puts weight on his sore foot. As a result, bones, joints, muscles, and tendons are being forced into unnatural positions so that the man can retain his balance when he is walking. The involvement of the bones, joints, and soft tissue spreads all the way up the leg, through the knees, the hips, and into the lower back, as the body strives to maintain equilibrium. Eventually a muscle or tendon will be strained or a joint will become inflamed, because bones and soft tissue around the joints will be pulled out of synch, and the man will feel pain all the way up into his spinal column, since, as the old song goes, the foot bone is eventually connected to the backbone—as is everything in between. The man now has aches and pains from his lower back all the way down to the callus on the bottom of his foot, where the problem originated. All that discomfort can make a man very unhappy, to the point where his mental and emotional well-being is adversely affected. All because of one little callus on the ball of his foot.

As I stated at the outset, foot disorders rarely place a person's life in jeopardy. However, they can create a fair bit of misery and dysfunction, so they ought not to be ignored to the extent they have been in the past. A well-informed general public will save a lot of aggravation and unnecessary visits to the doctor to repair problems that could have been resolved much more easily when they first arose.

The medical profession still has a long way to go to properly educate the public about foot problems. However, there is a change in the wind, and there are two major factors contributing to this increased awareness of proper foot care. The first of these is the boom in physical-fitness programs; the second is the fact that more people are living longer. The increase in the average age of the population means a natural increase in the circulatory and other problems affecting the aged, which create more foot disorders.

This book is not directed specifically at athletes and the older generation, but at the general public. However, since these two groups have been instrumental in awakening medical professionals to foot problems and the relationships between feet and other parts of the body, I want to touch briefly here on how they have contributed to the growth of foot research.

The Athlete's Foot
Athletes are particularly susceptible to foot problems because, as you will learn in Chapter Fourteen, certain physical activities place tremendous stresses on the foot. Athletes are generally quick to seek relief from their discomforts so that they can return to their favorite activities, and since many of the injuries they suffer are to the lower extremities, the feet are being examined far more closely than in the past. So, in a sense, the boom in physical fitness has brought the foot out of the closet and into the spotlight. As a result, research into the biomechanics of the foot and lower leg has become big

business. This will result not only in happier, healthier athletes, but in immense benefits to the general population, as foot specialists learn how to diagnose and correct foot disorders before they become severe.

For the past few years I have been involved with the S. C. Cooper Family Sports Medicine Clinic at Mount Sinai Hospital in Toronto. I am now seeing over seventy-five athletes a week with foot and related problems. One of the major benefits of the program at the Clinic, besides helping athletes heal, is the amount we have learned, from treating these patients, about the mechanics of the lower limbs, and how mechanical defects can affect everybody—not just athletes — and can also have an effect on other parts of the body.

Old Footage

The increasing number of older people in our modern society has also helped focus attention on the feet. Such people are very susceptible to certain conditions that affect their feet, either directly or indirectly: poor circulation in the lower extremities, reduced nerve function in the feet, reduced mobility, or simply the inability to see their feet clearly enough. Many older people cannot examine their feet or care for them properly because of failing eyesight or joint dysfunctions that prevent them from bending over. As a result, about sixty per cent of all my geriatric patients suffer from one or more fungal nails (see Chapter Ten) that go unnoticed unless they become painful or are spotted by a medical expert.

As I have just mentioned, older people are extremely prone to infections on their feet because of reduced circulation and nerve function, and for the same reasons they often cannot see or feel the condition until the infection has become acute. Calluses, corns, ingrown toenails, and other disorders go untreated until they have become extremely painful—occasionally because ulcers have formed beneath overlying irritated skin. The situation can be complicated if the older person is diabetic (see Chapter Eleven), because the disease contributes to poor circulation in the foot. If these conditions are allowed to develop, the complications could become quite serious. The infections that may result are often fuelled by over-the-counter or home remedies bought by older people in the mistaken belief that such items as corn-removers will relieve them of their discomforts.

The care of the feet of the aging was at best dismal well into the 1980s. But now that "grey power" has established a foothold and demanded equal rights, the overall health-care picture for this group should show improvement. As I have mentioned, one of the results will be increased interest in foot care, since such a large percentage of the geriatric population suffers from assorted foot disorders that could deleteriously affect their lives.

Foot Fantasies: Misconceptions and Old Wives' Tales
Although we can thank athletes and the older generation for the rapidly expanding interest in foot-care research and treatment, we still have to consider that most of the patients I see these days for the first time know very little about what can go wrong with their feet and how to care for them properly. Many of them have been misinformed, either by old wives' tales or by well-meaning, competent medical professionals, who, however, lack specific expertise in proper foot care. Others have absolutely no concept of how the foot functions — the *biomechanics* of the foot in motion. The sad fact is that many foot problems are ignored or made worse by sheer ignorance and are easily avoidable. I believe that by the time a patient has completed proper treatment for a foot disorder, he or she should be able to resume a normal life-style quickly, knowing that the problem ought not to recur if the proper precautions are taken.

Most of the misinformation people receive involves the more common foot complaints—corns, calluses, bunions, plantar warts, and ingrown toenails. Other common misconceptions occur concerning footwear and foot surgery. Parents often panic needlessly—and mistakenly—when they believe that baby's first steps are abnormal.

Sadly, one of the major misconceptions involves the joints of the feet—for that matter, all the joints in the body. I am referring to the condition called *osteoarthritis*. I agree with many of my medical colleagues who argue forcefully that osteoarthritis is not a disease, but a normal wear-and-tear process that is often accelerated because of a mechanical fault that affects certain joints in a particular part of the body. Osteoarthritis is occasionally mis-diagnosed because its symptoms can mimic those of other disorders. But, regardless of how accurate the diagnosis may be, the mention of the word arthritis can strike terror into the minds of its victims, who believe that they will be racked with terrible and unavoidable pain in their joints for the rest of their lives. I hope that by the time you finish reading this book you will understand the process of arthritis much better, and be less fearful of the disorder. Many arthritic conditions can be controlled by correcting the biomechanical fault that initially caused a joint to wear down. The joints may not necessarily be in the feet, but foot problems can subject the joint to undue stress, leading to breakdown.

The Leaning Tower of Pisa Syndrome

I spoke earlier of the fact that a foot problem can affect other parts of the body, and I have just mentioned the misconceptions involving osteoarthritis. Because the disorder is a wear-and-tear process of the joints, it can be accelerated by a situation in which a biomechanical foot fault places undue stress on various parts of the lower extremities. Although it is most often athletes who seek immediate relief from discomfort in their knees, hips, lower back, and other areas of the lower limbs, all segments of the population can be afflicted by such disorders, which are either directly or indirectly caused by foot problems. I call this situation the "Leaning Tower of Pisa Syndrome".

The foundation of the famous Leaning Tower of Pisa is not perfectly balanced. Therefore the tower leans—a trifle more each year, according to expert measurements. While an edifice does not experience pain—it may only eventually collapse—your body certainly can if your foundation is not level and solid. Like the Tower, your entire structure can wind up out of kilter. When this occurs, musculoskeletal problems can arise, usually from the lower spine downwards, as the bones, muscles, tendons, and other soft tissue in the lower extremities struggle to keep the body in balance. This added strain may eventually force the joints—for example, those in the lower back, in the hips, in the knees—out of kilter. A joint that is not allowed to function normally will eventually begin to wear out. As you will discover in Chapter Three, when that happens bone will begin to rub against bone, and arthritic pain will occur.

Although I do not specifically treat people with low-back, knee, or hip pain, my orthopedic colleagues and I have successfully dealt with disorders in these areas by correcting foot abnormalities. However, I caution the reader against thinking that back, hip, or knee problems are commonly caused or exacerbated by bad feet. As far as back patients are concerned, I see them only after they have gone through rigorous examination by back specialists who have exhausted all conventional, conservative steps.

I will have much more to say about the Leaning Tower of Pisa Syndrome and how it affects certain parts of the body in Chapter Three. It is important to remember in the meantime that this syndrome can be responsible for many cases of arthritis and other joint disorders.

Fear and Communication
I have already mentioned the problem about misconceptions concerning care of the feet. This problem is often compounded, particularly when common conditions, such as osteoarthritis, are involved, by the inability of the patient and the doctor to communicate.

When I began contemplating writing this book, one of the problems I wished to address was that of medical "miscommunication"— a combination of misinformation and a lack of understanding between medical professionals and their patients.

During my first year at the school of podiatry, when I was an impressionable young student, a professor emphasized in one of his early lectures that some of the most common questions we will hear in our offices will concern fear of the unknown. The patient knows only that his or her feet hurt terribly, but does not know why. Will he or she ever be able to walk normally again? Is the problem serious?

I get these questions from at least two or three new patients every day. It is the fear of not knowing the cause of their discomfort, or the severity of the condition, that causes them the most grief. As the same professor emphasized to his new students: If a patient does not understand the nature of the discomfort, the misery will be compounded to the point where the entire body and psyche are adversely affected.

Sad to say, however, many podiatrists and other medical professionals often conduct themselves as if the last thing they want to contribute to the relationship with their patients is understandable, factual information. A typical conversation between patient and doctor might go as follows:

PATIENT: Doc, my foot hurts terribly in the front, on the bottom. (Patient points to the ball of his/her foot.)

DOCTOR: (Upon examining foot) Hmmm. ("Hmmm" is one of the first words learned in medical school. It immediately establishes fear and doubt in the patient, while at the same time providing the doctor with a few precious moments to determine exactly what he ought to tell the new patient. For taciturn and/or condescending doctors the expression serves to keep an undemanding patient in the dark.)

PATIENT: What's wrong, Doc? Is it serious?

DOCTOR: (After completing his examination of the foot) You have metatarsalgia.

PATIENT: (Wondering if he/she will ever be able to walk normally again) Oh my God!

After the doctor has finally revived the patient, he condescends to explain that *metatarsalgia* is nothing more than a pain in the foot between the ankle and the toes—precisely what the patient had told the doctor when first questioned. Only if the patient had been a student of ancient languages would he/she have been able to figure out the meaning of the long word before the doctor explained it.

Metatarsalgia is a foreign word belonging to the language known as "medicalese". Approximately fifty thousand new words of medicalese are taught to students in medical school, and, if they do not continue to constantly use these words, they will tend to forget them, just like any foreign language. A foreign tongue can often instill fear in a person unfamiliar with it, and build a sense of power in the linguist. As a group, doctors are no different from linguists, and patients are often more easily cowed by words they cannot understand than others are. Hence, a chasm can develop between patient and doctor that may never be bridged, to the detriment of both parties.

One of my patients' greatest fears is "arthritis"—a word doctors regularly use when dealing with people suffering from joint pain. I would like to have a dollar for every time a person is told by a doctor that a lower limb or back pain is indicative of arthritis and that very little can be done to be rid of the condition, other than taking Aspirins and moving to Arizona.

As I have already stated, one of the myths I intend to dispel in this book is the belief that *osteoarthritis* (osteo, "bone"; arthro, "joint"; itis, "inflammation of") is a disease about which nothing can be done. (There are, of course, other types of arthritis, which I will discuss in Chapter Eleven, that are indeed diseases.)

Before my medical colleagues begin jumping all over me for accusing them of being solely responsible for a communication gap between doctors and patients, let me say that the problem is usually a two-way street. Patients often do not know what to ask a doctor—or do not want to hear the truth—and even a doctor with the best intentions, who is an able communicator, will find it hard to get across the facts. I hope that a careful reading of this book will help patients ask the right questions when they visit a medical practitioner for a foot problem. I am not too sure, however, what to do with those patients who refuse to hear the truth.

Communication between doctor and patient can also be disastrous when neither manages to communicate precisely what he or she wants or expects. A typical conversation might go as follows:

PATIENT: Doc, there is something sticking out on the side of my big toe.

DOCTOR: Hmmm. You have hallux valgus. (This is medicalese for "bunion", but the patient does not know this.)

PATIENT: Doc, I can't wear my shoes any more because my foot hurts so much. And it's so hard to find shoes that are larger and look good. I've got big feet to begin with. (What the patient probably means is that he/she wants to be able to wear stylish shoes, whatever the cost.)

DOCTOR: (Understanding only that the patient's foot hurts) Well, I can certainly operate to remove the problem and relieve the pain. It won't be too difficult, and you won't be out of action for very long.

The patient believes that surgery will enable him or her to fit into comfortable and stylish shoes, so the operation is booked. At this point, the patient and the doctor are on totally different wave-lengths: the doctor has no idea that the patient is expecting cosmetic surgery, and the patient has no idea of what bunion surgery involves. After the operation the patient will discover that, once the foot has healed, the uncomfortable but stylish shoes will still be too tight because the size of the foot has remained the same. The surgeon has removed a bunion; he has not radically altered the shape of the patient's foot. The patient will also learn for the first time that he/she will probably be required to wear an insert in the shoe to prevent the recurrence of the bunion. The patient will suffer from post-bunion depression because he or she had unreal expectations; the doctor will be irritated by the patient's complaints about the operation being a total failure. So, nobody wins, because the rules of the game were never established.

As the patient referred to above sadly discovered, it is important for a person facing surgery to understand basically (not necessarily in great detail) how the operation will be performed, what it can accomplish, the amount of discomfort involved after the operation, and the time it will take for him or her to recover. I intend to explain in this book how certain common types of foot surgery are performed — for example, how corns, bunions, and ingrown toenails are removed — so that you will understand, if you ever have to undergo any of these procedures, that most of them are relatively minor, can be done on an out-patient basis either in a hospital or in a doctor's office, and do not require lengthy, painful periods of recuperation. My patients respond to the thought of foot surgery with far less anxiety when they are fully informed, and they tend to recuperate far more quickly—with fewer, if any, complications.

What's My Line
I trust that by now I have convinced you that there is a need for the general public to know a great deal more about their feet in order to allay fears and misconceptions. Now, just where do I fit into the picture?

Podiatrists are not doctors with foot fetishes. They may be doctors who "bill the foot", as a wisecracking patient once joked, but they are much more than that. A podiatrist specializes in caring for the lower extremities of the body—not just the area from the heel to the toe, but generally from the top of the ankle on down. Specializing in feet may not seem so appetizing, but medical professionals often focus on a specific disease or a part of the body because they or family members or friends suffer from specific ailments. These professionals are seeking ways to relieve the discomforts from which they or loved ones suffer. While I was growing up, my mother constantly complained about her bad feet. When her feet ached, her mood was adversely affected, and that meant misery for the rest of the family. For her sake—and mine—I wanted to help her; so, I became a podiatrist.

A podiatrist goes through an educational process that is similar to that of a medical doctor (M.D.): three years of pre-medical studies at a recognized university in North America, followed by four years of training at one of six colleges of podiatric medicine in the United States. (There are none in Canada at this time.) Most graduates of these colleges then take at least one year of residency in an accredited hospital before going into private practice.

Although I cannot hang out my shingle as an M.D., as a podiatrist (D.P.M.) I am a respected member of the medical community in Toronto. I work out of two large downtown teaching hospitals where I enjoy rights accorded to M.D. staff members and perform foot surgery. I am particularly fortunate, however, because podiatrists have not yet been fully accepted by all members of the medical establishment in Canada and the United States, although the situation is rapidly changing and we hope to soon enjoy equal status with other American and Canadian medical associations.

Since I practise with—and have great faith in—my M.D. colleagues, and since they, in turn, have shown confidence in me, I have no intention in this book of taking the medical profession to task. What I would like to emphasize is that, be they family practitioners or specialists, most M.D.s, by the very nature of their medical training, do not receive sufficient education about the biomechanics of the foot, about how bad feet can affect the rest of the body, about the causes and prevention of foot disorders, or about how to treat abnormal foot conditions when they arise. They are normally too busy treating patients with serious, often life-threatening disorders—malignancies, cardiovascular diseases, or severe emotional conditions, to name a few.

This means that the foot is often the most neglected part of the body, because foot diseases or disorders are rarely, if ever, life-threatening, unless gangrene or severe infection is allowed to spread up into the leg and then into the rest of the body.

Some doctors tend to ignore their patients' feet completely. How often have you had a complete physical in which you were told to leave on your socks? How many mothers have dragged their young children to the doctor to complain that their child's feet were either toeing in or toeing out, and were told that the child would outgrow the condition—only to find about ten years down the road that the problem still exists? How many runners with knee, hip, or low-back pain have been told to stop running by medical professionals who were unaware that the discomfort may have been caused by a foot problem that could easily have been corrected? We have seen many runners at our sports-medicine clinics who have been able to resume their activity after having a knee, hip, or low-back problem eliminated by treatment of a foot dysfunction.

It has been estimated by medical researchers that about eighty per cent of the population of "advanced" countries will suffer from back pain at one time or another. I have already mentioned that I believe the same to hold true for foot problems. There are thousands of doctors in the world who specialize in backs. Why does the same not hold true for foot doctors? There is also a spate of books written by medical professionals for people with back problems, but almost none for those with foot problems. The more I thought about these facts, the greater my desire became to help educate a generally unaware public about their feet. I would like to share with the reader the experience and knowledge I have gained over the past decade, so that as many people as possible may avoid the years of misery which my mother, among others, suffered needlessly.

However, before you get the idea that I am writing this book merely to pat myself on the back, and to claim that I and other podiatrists are infallible when it comes to treating foot problems, let me tell you that I have seen a few cases that have left me shaking my head in bewilderment.

As much as I love to debunk old wives' tales about treatments for various foot problems, I must admit that I have had more than one patient who has gotten rid of plantar warts by spitting on them, or rubbing them with a potato that was then left in the kitchen cupboard for a month—after all the conventional forms of treatment that I had prescribed had failed.

One of my patients with a sense of humor is always reminding me that doctors do not always have the right answers, even though they may always have glib ones. Two of his jokes come to mind.

A limping man who had one leg shorter than the other asked his doctor what the doctor would do under the circumstances. The doctor answered, "I'd limp as well."

The other joke concerns the man who was examined by a podiatrist for a wide variety of foot complaints and demanded to know what he could do when he left the doctor's office. "Take a taxi," the doctor replied.

Forgive the humor, but I have come to realize that health-care books have to be both entertaining and a bit controversial, as well as factual, to have a lasting, favorable impact. So I certainly do not apologize for trying to be entertaining, since humor often helps to hit home the serious messages. As for controversy, I have already stated that I do not intend to blow my own horn at the expense of other medical professionals by contradicting their beliefs or admonishing them for their lack of knowledge of the foot. But I specialize in feet; most of my medical colleagues do not. As a result, a few of them may take exception to some of my opinions because they are not aware of the state of the art in foot care. However, we usually work well as a team—I see their patients with foot problems, and consult with them when their expertise is required to help my patients. Keep in mind, though, that I am neither a magician nor a miracle-worker; on the other hand, I know a lot about feet, and I would like to share some of that knowledge with you.

Three Little Words

Although I have promised to do my best in this book to avoid medicalese, there are three technical words that will crop up repeatedly: *biomechanics*, *pronation*, and *orthotics*. I will define these terms precisely in Chapter Three. However, a brief explanation of them may be in order here in case you intend to skim through or scan the book before reading it in detail.

Biomechanics refers to the study of human motion. For our purposes, we will look more specifically at the biomechanics of the foot and lower leg. When the biomechanics of our stride is abnormal when we walk, run, or do other activities, we run into problems. The most common of these problems is abnormal *pronation* and involves an abnormal rolling of the weight-bearing foot from the outside in. As you will discover in later chapters, pronation can be responsible for a whole host of foot and lower-limb disorders. One of the ways of treating the pronation syndrome is with *orthotics*—inserts that fit into shoes to enable weight to be distributed properly throughout the foot during the time it is on the ground and is bearing that weight.

I suspect that if you ever have a foot problem that takes you to a foot specialist for relief, you will hear at least one, if not all three, of these terms. If you understand the meaning of the words, you will know that the doctor is not throwing medicalese at you to mask a terrible disease or painful treatment. In all likelihood he will be telling you that your condition is not serious, and is easily treatable without the need for invasive action, like surgery. And if you understand these three words, you will capture the essence of this book, because the majority of patients I see in my private practice and at the clinics with which I am affiliated have biomechanical foot faults that most commonly involve pronation, and at least part of the treatment for a condition caused by abnormal pronation of a foot may involve the insertion of an orthotic device into the shoe to correct the biomechanical disorder.

2

The Anatomy of the Foot

Foot Faults?

It never ceases to amaze me how so many of my patients continually complain about the size and shape of their feet—they are either too big or too small, too wide or too narrow, too thick or too thin, or just plain fat and ugly. I have never understood why so many people hate their feet, or the feet of others, and I probably never will.

The only person I ever met who thought his feet were beautiful was my Uncle Harold. One evening, during a formal cocktail party at his home, he summoned me to his library, sat down, removed his shoes and socks, and put his feet up on his desk. He then pointed to them with the big fat cigar he was smoking at the time.

"Is there something wrong, Uncle?" I asked him with concern. I assumed he had a problem and was seeking medical advice.

Uncle Harold chewed on his cigar for a minute, then said proudly, "Beeeautiful, aren't they. I just wanted to show you, since you probably see only ugly ones in your office."

As I stood momentarily speechless, Uncle Harold put his shoes and socks back on, got up, and returned to the party. He may have been slightly inebriated, but to me he was a breath of fresh air. I only wish my patients would feel the same way about their feet, rather than constantly running them down.

While many people simply do not like the shape of their feet, others complain regularly about how dysfunctional the foot is. A few months ago I was sitting in the doctors' lounge at a hospital where I practise, waiting my turn in the operating room. I was joined by a medical colleague, an obstetrician, who asked me, during the course of our conversation, why I chose feet as my specialty. I was about to suggest that the question might be more appropriately asked of a proctologist when he launched into a dissertation as to why the foot was the most disgusting part of the human body, a part that "most definitely ought to be left at home when going out on a date."

"Just what is so disgusting about the human foot?" I asked.

"The size, shape, overall design, everything," he replied smugly. "It's total imperfection. But I guess that's why you chose podiatry. You must be making a fortune treating all those problems caused by bad feet."

I thought about his remarks for a few moments, then I asked how he would have better designed the foot for its tasks.

The obstetrician took a pad and pencil and drew a 3"-by-6" block. "Simple," he said, and shrugged.

"Just a minute," I replied. "The foot has to act as a lever to propel the body. A block can't do that."

My colleague took his pencil and added what he described as a hinge joint near the front of his block.

I then pointed out to him that his structure was basically inflexible and could not turn in or out. He thought for a moment, then drew another hinge joint at the rear end of the block. But he was obviously not pleased.

He became even more annoyed when I complained about the lack of a balance mechanism in his foot, a lack that would make any movement most awkward, despite his two hinges. He began chopping up the front of his model foot, and when he had finished, it appeared as if he had given the block five toes. He scowled, then glowered at me as he examined the results, but he was saved further discomfort by the beeping of his pager. His patient was about to deliver, and I was not surprised to learn that the baby elected to emerge feet first, to remind him of our discussion.

So, my patients dislike their "ugly" feet, and my medical colleagues often view the foot with disdain. All the more reason for me to put the foot up on a pedestal, and to convince people to put esthetics aside and learn how the foot functions and why it is shaped the way it is.

What's A-foot?

A foot is more than just a strangely shaped thing at the end of a leg. It is, or ought to be, the most dependable form of transportation you have, and it may often be an excellent barometer of your general physical condition.

You may imagine, if you wish, that your body is a Rolls-Royce, and that your feet are the wheels. In fact, athletes often prefer to call their lower extremities "wheels". If your "wheels" are out of alignment, your total performance suffers. Conversely, trouble elsewhere in your body can manifest itself in your feet.

We will return to the analogy of your body as a machine later, but first I want to illustrate, verbally and with diagrams, the anatomy of the foot—the bones and joints, the muscles and tendons, the ligaments, the cartilages, the veins and arteries, and the nerves. Once I have dealt with all the integral parts of the foot, I will proceed, in the next chapter, to illustrate how they all work together to enable you to walk, run, dance, play, or do whatever else you wish.

A Quick, Painless Course in Anatomy

Those in favor of complete metrication of our measurement systems will be pleased to learn that a foot, ugly or beautiful, is not always twelve inches. Foot size in a normal, healthy adult can range from 4½ inches long by 3 inches wide to 17 inches long by 7 inches wide. In most cases feet are generally made to order for a particular body shape and size. A common complaint I hear from exceptionally tall women is the difficulty they have in finding esthetically pleasing shoes to fit what they consider to be huge, unattractive feet. However, these women would look very silly with size 5 or 6 feet. Moreover, they would not be able to properly balance themselves, and would probably blow over in high winds. I advise these women to complain to shoe designers and manufacturers, not to their fate, for satisfaction.

I do not wish to bore you with endless fine details and medical terminology that will only confuse and discourage you, so I will try to keep the heavy stuff to a basic minimum, while at the same time providing you with enough information to enable you to understand how the foot functions and why it so often causes you pain and discomfort.

I promise to do my best to avoid, or at least explain, "medicalese".

I always hated learning new languages, and medical terminology was no exception. If you want everything in proper medicalese, I suggest that you buy yourself a copy of *Gray's Anatomy*.

Medical experts have divided the foot into three distinct parts: the *forefoot*, from the toes to the base of the metatarsals (the five bones that connect the midfoot and rearfoot bones to the toe bones); the *midfoot*, including the cuneiforms, the cuboid, and the navicular bones (see Diagram 2:1); and the *rearfoot*, including the *talus* (ankle

DIAGRAM 2:1
The Three Major Sections of the Foot

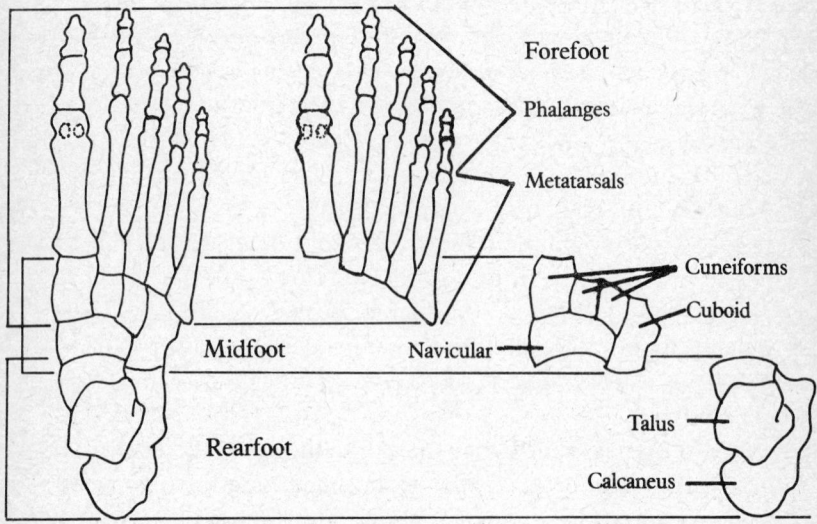

bone) and the *calcaneus* (heel bone). Many people refer to the "ball" of the foot, and the "arch", without really knowing exactly where they are located. The ball is considered to be in the forefoot—on the bottom of the foot, under the metatarsal heads. The arch is generally considered to be in the midfoot area, which is shown in this diagram.

It is an interesting fact, at least to me, that over ninety-five per cent of all foot surgery is done on the forefoot. I will explain why in various chapters throughout the book.

Dem Bones

A quarter of all the bones in the human body are in the feet. The normal foot has twenty-six bones of varying sizes and shapes (see Diagram 2:2) plus two sesamoids. However, it is not uncommon for

DIAGRAM 2:2
The Bones of the Foot and Positions of Accessory Ossicles

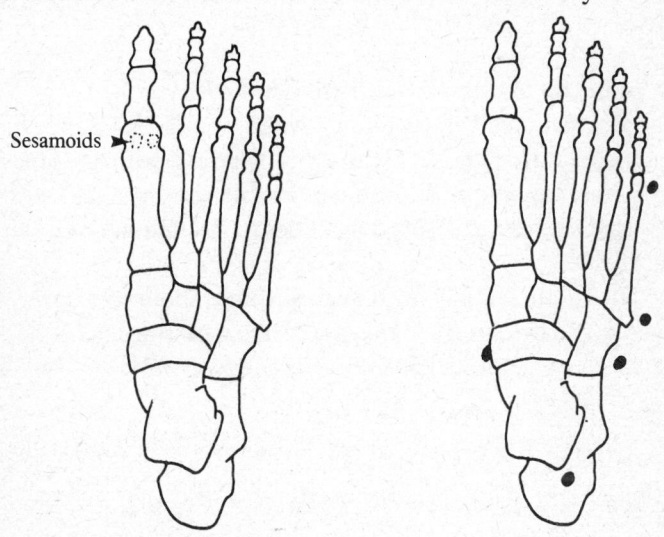

Twenty-six Bones of the Foot, plus   Sites of Accessory
the Sesamoids   Ossicles

a person to have extra small bones called *accessory ossicles*. These extra bones seldom cause any trouble, and are thought to be hereditary. In Diagram 2:2 you can see the six most common areas of the foot where these accessory ossicles are found.

It would be a medical rarity for anyone to have too few bones in the foot. My day would be complete if such a foot were to enter my office. Most doctors I know love to see benign, but unusual, cases from time to time, and I am no exception.

Bones and biomechanics go together, as you will learn in the following chapter. Getting back to our analogy of the body as a machine, you know that when one cog in a wheel is misshapen, the machinery will malfunction. The same holds true for the foot when one of its bones is defective. An abnormal bone can lead to a biomechanical fault. But before we get to biomechanical details, we have to examine other parts of the foot—the joints, and the soft tissues that hold the bones and joints in place and facilitate their movement; the soft tissues, such as muscles, tendons, cartilages, and ligaments; the supply system that lubricates and nourishes the bones and soft tissues; and the electrical, or nerve, system that transmits signals to and from the brain.

Joints

Two or more bones that come together *articulate* to form a joint. We hear a great deal about joints when we discuss arthritis and cartilage problems, and they can be a terrible pain at times. But without joints we would be quite inflexible, because most of them move, at least slightly, to allow our bodies to assume different motions and postures.

The joint in the foot you probably think about the most is the ankle joint, which connects the lower part of the leg to the back of the foot (see Diagram 2:3). It is a hinge-type joint; in a sense,

DIAGRAM 2:3
Joints of the Foot and Ankle

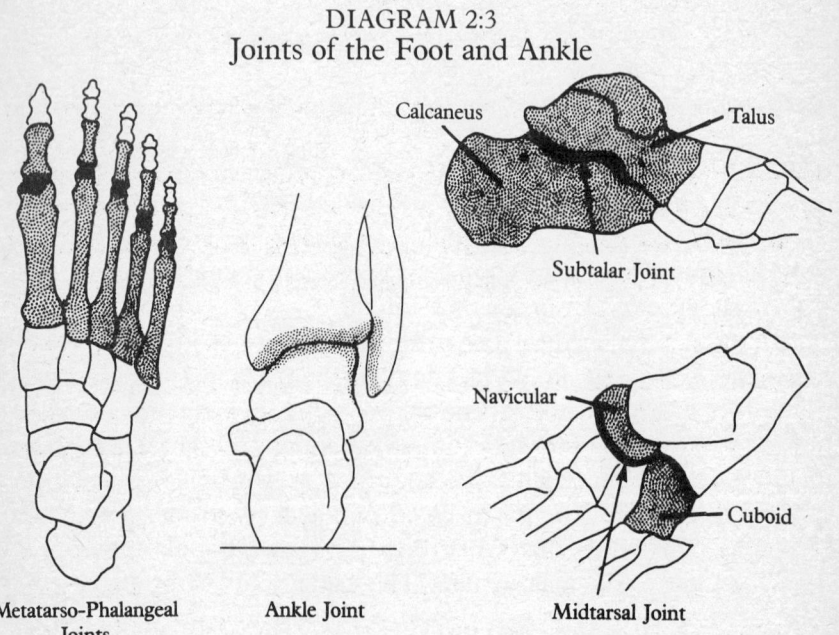

Calcaneus

Talus

Subtalar Joint

Navicular

Cuboid

Metatarso-Phalangeal
Joints

Ankle Joint

Midtarsal Joint

the motion in the area resembles that of a door opening. When the ankle joint is damaged, walking or running becomes a problem, because of the pain that occurs when weight is placed on the foot. A person's gait can become exaggerated as he or she attempts to compensate and force most of the weight onto the other foot during the walking cycle. As a result, the biomechanics of both feet can be adversely affected.

However, the most crucial joint affecting the biomechanics of the foot during walking or running is the *subtalar* (see Diagram 2:3). It comprises three different *articulations* (where bones come together) between the top surface of the heel bone and the bottom surface of the ankle bone. As you will see in the following chapter, when a person pronates abnormally, the subtalar joint does not move as it should. If this occurs, problems can develop throughout the foot.

The *midtarsal* joint, in the arch area of the foot (see Diagram 2:3), works together with the subtalar joint to help the foot compensate for a biomechanical fault, particularly the type that is temporary. This could occur when a person is walking or running on an uneven terrain, or when there is a change in upper-body motion—for example, when an athlete or a dancer assumes an unusual position. When the subtalar and midtarsal joints are unable to compensate adequately for a biomechanical fault that is fairly long-lasting, the result could be a foot disorder.

It is not likely that a person will suffer from subtalar or midtarsal joint pain to any great extent. There is one other joint in the foot, though, that can cause excruciating pain at times. It is the *metatarso-phalangeal* joint that is formed by the articulation of the head of each metatarsal bone, situated in the ball area of the foot, and the end of each *phalanx* (the large bone in the toes). This joint can be seen in Diagram 2:3.

For reasons that I will describe in subsequent chapters, the big-toe joint—where the *proximal phalanx* (the big toe-bone of the first, or great, toe) and the metatarsal head come together—often accepts the brunt of unequal weight distribution that a biomechanical fault inflicts on a foot. As a result, this joint is subjected to a lot of added wear and tear that makes it susceptible to osteoarthritis and similar conditions. Although *gout* may affect the big-toe joint, it is not caused by a biomechanical problem. It is a disease that can be controlled by proper medication and diet, as you will discover in Chapter Eleven.

Obviously there are many other joints in the foot, although our major concern in this book is the four joints mentioned above, because they are the ones that most affect, and are affected by, biomechanical foot faults. However, it is not uncommon to have problems with the *interphalangeal* joints between the *phalanges*, or toe bones, in the various toes. (There are two bones that comprise the big toe, and three bones in all the other toes.) When I discuss forefoot pain in Chapter Six, I will deal with conditions that can affect these phalangeal joints.

Muscle-Bound

There are nineteen individual muscles in the foot and lower leg. If you examine Diagrams 2:4 and 2:5 carefully, you will learn the major muscles, and how they interconnect with other parts of the foot to help move it. I assume that you all understand the vital role of muscles in the body, so that I can avoid a tedious explanation of their functions. When muscles are overstressed, or are otherwise abnormal, they can affect the biomechanics of the foot, because they

DIAGRAM 2:4
Layers of Dorsal Muscles

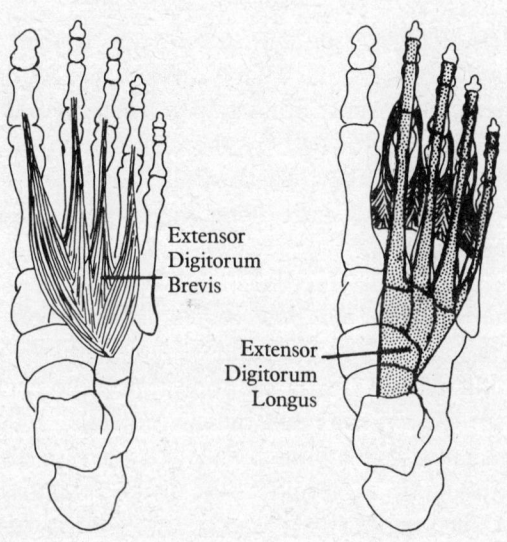

Extensor
Digitorum
Brevis

Extensor
Digitorum
Longus

DIAGRAM 2:5
Layers of Plantar Muscles and Tendons

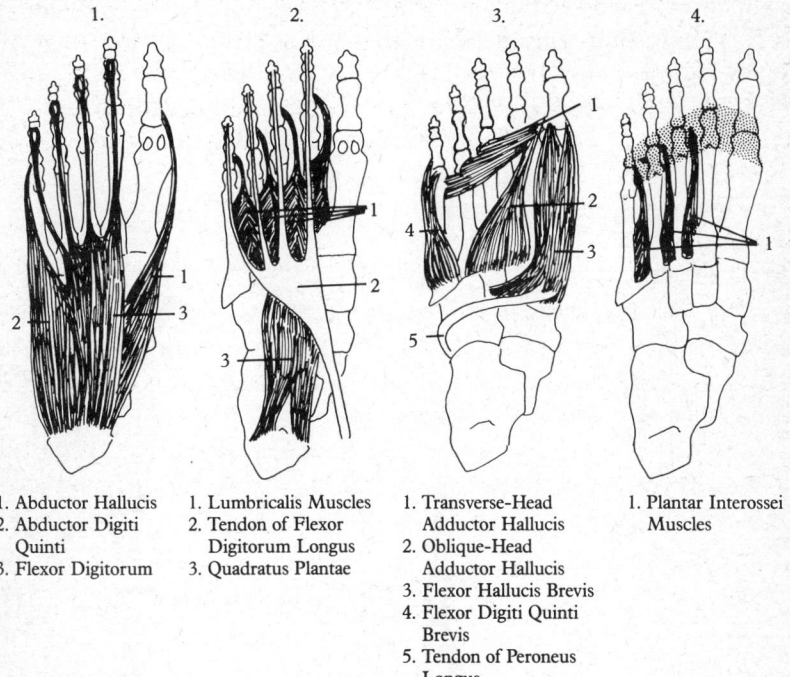

1. Abductor Hallucis
2. Abductor Digiti
   Quinti
3. Flexor Digitorum

1. Lumbricalis Muscles
2. Tendon of Flexor
   Digitorum Longus
3. Quadratus Plantae

1. Transverse-Head
   Adductor Hallucis
2. Oblique-Head
   Adductor Hallucis
3. Flexor Hallucis Brevis
4. Flexor Digiti Quinti
   Brevis
5. Tendon of Peroneus
   Longus

1. Plantar Interossei
   Muscles

can pull tendons and bones out of place, and irritate joints. Conversely, muscles can be injured as a result of a bone defect. I will discuss damage to particular muscles of the foot in great detail in subsequent chapters. I will also describe, particularly in the chapters dealing with sports medicine, how muscles in the leg can affect, or be affected by, the biomechanics of the feet.

Tendons

Tendons attach muscles to bones (see Diagram 2:6). Actually, they are extensions of muscles, and are tough, whitish cords that are somewhat elastic and flexible. When a muscle has been stretched to its maximum potential, the force of the stretch is transferred to the tendon. The tendon itself may then be overstretched, and this situation results in *tendonitis*, inflammation of the tendon.

Ligaments

Ligaments are thick, inelastic, but flexible structures that support and surround joints, holding bone to bone (see Diagram 2:6). When an ankle is twisted or a big toe is stubbed, the cause of all the discomfort and swelling is usually a ligament that has been overstretched, or somewhat torn.

DIAGRAM 2:6
Ligaments, Tendons, and Cartilage of the Foot and Leg

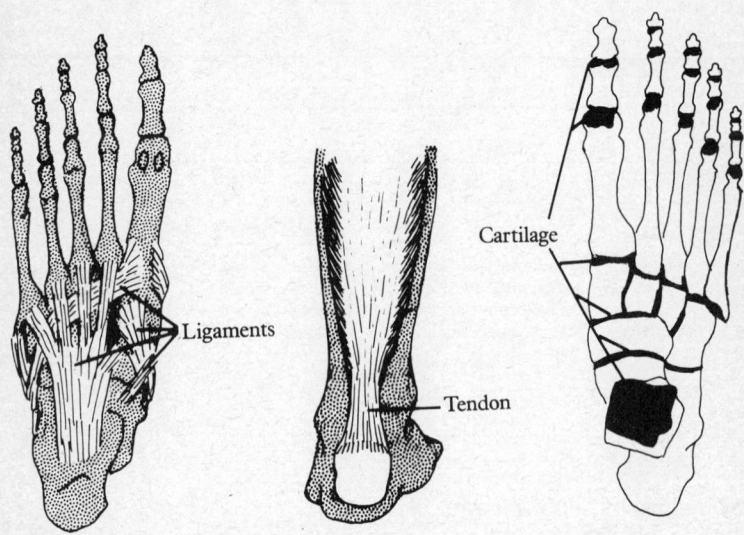

Cartilage

Cartilage is dense connective tissue that serves as a lining on the ends of bones where they meet to form joints (see Diagram 2:6). If you eat a chicken drumstick, you will notice the white gristle lining the end of the bone. That white gristle is cartilage.

Cartilage provides smooth surfaces between bones. Without cartilage, your body would literally grind to a halt. Your joints would make a terrible racket when you moved, as bone would grind against bone. You would also be in terrible pain from the inflammation in the joints caused by the bones grinding together.

In Circulation

There are two main arteries that supply the feet with the necessary blood supply: the *dorsalis pedis* artery and the *posterior tibial* artery (see Diagram 2:7). These major arteries spread oxygenated blood

DIAGRAM 2:7
Arteries and Veins

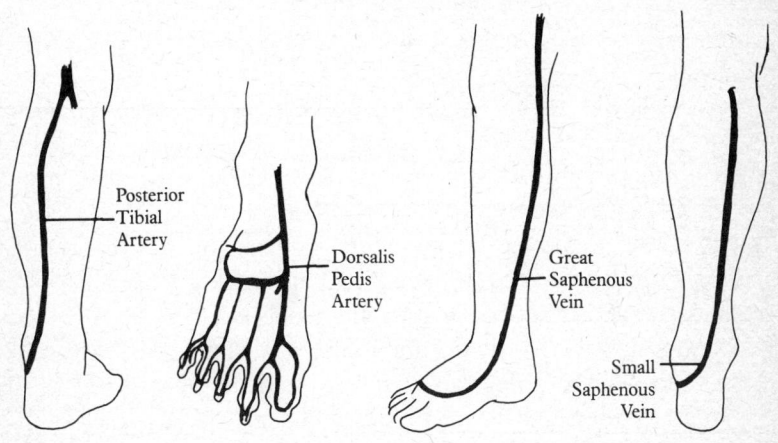

via smaller arterioles to the many tissues of the feet. A failure to supply life-supporting oxygen contained in the red blood cells by the arterial system could result in serious problems.

Because, in the human body, the major foot arteries are the farthest away from the heart, many circulatory problems will first manifest themselves in the feet. Two examples would be *arteriosclerosis* (hardening of the arteries) and *atherosclerosis* (a build-up of plaque inside the arteries, leading to subsequent blockage of the arteries).

We all know that veins are vessels that return used blood to the heart and lungs for regeneration—for nutrients and oxygen—after the blood's supply of oxygen has been used up to nourish the tissues of the body. There are two sets of veins that return blood from the lower extremities to the heart and lungs. The *superficial* veins that run close to the surface of the skin and remove spent (deoxygenated) blood from the feet to the heart and lungs are the *great saphenous* (the longest vein in the body, running up the big-toe side of the foot on the inside of the leg) and the *small saphenous* (which runs on the outside part of the foot and up the back of the leg). The deep veins that run farther below the surface of the skin arc the *anterior tibial* and the *posterior tibial*. The positioning of all the above-mentioned veins can be seen in Diagram 2:7. Incidentally, it is the great saphenous vein that heart surgeons sometimes dissect for use in bypass surgery.

Obviously there are tiny auxiliary veins (*venuoles*) that are the opposite of arterioles. They pick up used blood and deliver it to the larger veins for the journey up to the heart and lungs.

Capillaries are the cross-over links between the arterioles and the venuoles.

People with circulatory problems in their lower extremities often complain of swollen ankles, a condition that worsens after a long day on one's feet, or after a lengthy airplane flight. A majority of such problems, including varicose veins, are related to poor *venous* (vein) function in the feet. Treatments do exist for such conditions, and they will be described in detail in Chapter Eleven.

Podiatrists, and other medical professionals who are on their toes, will examine the feet of their patients for any changes in skin color, texture, and temperature. Such changes can be tip-offs to certain circulatory problems that will be described in Chapter Eleven. But I will tell you now that it would not be wise for you to try and make any diagnoses yourself. You might mistakenly decide that one of your toes looked and felt funny, and that this was probably indicative of serious cardiovascular disease.

You Have Your Nerves

We should all know that nerves supply feeling to a particular part of the body, and the foot is no different. It has four major nerves that provide you with many weird and wonderful sensations. These four nerves—the *posterior tibial*, the *superficial peroneal*, the *deep peroneal*, and the *sural*—can be identified in Diagram 2:8.

Nerve problems in the foot are commonly related to *compression* syndromes—that is, a nerve is being pinched or squeezed. For example, an improperly fitting shoe can put so much pressure on a nerve that the area around the nerve swells. This causes *nerve entrapment*, which in turn can lead to pain and numbness, and occasionally to a strange, seemingly unrelated discomfort that I call "enigmatic" pain. There are also nerve disorders in other parts of the body—for example, *sciatica*—that can have manifestations in the

DIAGRAM 2:8
Nerves of the Foot and Leg

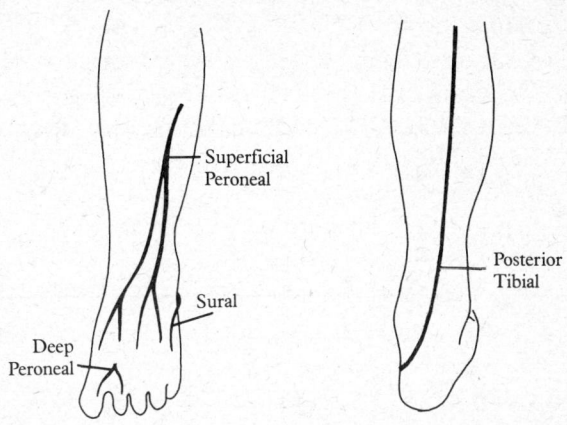

feet. These and other nerve diseases that affect the lower extremities will be discussed in various chapters throughout the book.

Functions of the Foot

Now that we know the roles of the major components of the foot, we ought to briefly examine the functions of the foot before we proceed to the chapter on biomechanics. It is important to know what the foot does to be able to understand why its proper mechanical range of motions is so vital in keeping a person on an even keel when walking or running.

First, the mobile foot helps you adapt to certain ground surfaces. If you have trouble adapting from walking or running on hard, soft, wet, or dry surfaces, you may often be falling on your face. The foot functions much as the tires on a car do to assure a smooth, safe ride on various terrains.

Secondly, the foot is a rigid lever that propels the body forward—and in other directions. If you had a block for a foot, as my obstetrician colleague suggested, you would have great difficulty maneuvering your body in any direction.

Thirdly, the foot is a shock-absorber that absorbs most of the shock to the body while you are on your feet. Unless the foot performed this function, other shock-absorbing areas of the body, such as the knees and the spinal column, would be under extreme stress that would cause early wear-and-tear on their joints.

The fact that the human foot accomplishes these three feats is actually quite amazing. As one of my professors said to me years ago, "It's not the problems of the foot that intrigue me as much as what the foot is capable of withstanding during the course of a normal lifetime." So, with all due respect to my obstetrician colleague, I intend to prove to you that nature did not design such a monstrosity for a lower appendage after all.

3
The Biomechanics of the Foot and Lower Leg

Introduction
I know that the following discussion of the biomechanics of the lower extremities may seem complicated. However, it is important for you to have a decent grasp of the topic, because biomechanical faults account for an overwhelming number of foot problems, and a significant amount of the discomfort that is felt from the lower back down to the foot.

To make life easier, I have simplified the details almost to a fault, because an exhaustive examination of the mechanics of walking or running would require extensive knowledge in various related fields—for example, in medicine, in physics, in kinestheology, and in ergonomics. Also, a complete treatment of the subject would take about eight hundred pages. What I have tried to do is to help you understand how your foot moves, and how certain disorders of the foot and lower limbs can be caused either directly or indirectly by a biomechanical fault. You will need this information to be able to understand much of the material in the following chapters.

Definition
For the purposes of this book, I would define *biomechanics* as the study of the mechanical laws of human motion, specifically movement of the lower leg and foot.

The graceful motions of a ballet dancer, or a runner in full, fluid stride, could provide suitable examples of essentially flawless biomechanics in action. Perhaps the prime example of perfect biomechanics would be a champion racehorse in full flight down the homestretch, but this is a book about humans, not horses, so we shall not dwell on this analogy.

Biomechanics Research

It is only within the past fifteen or so years that podiatrists have joined the forefront of researchers seeking to understand abnormal walking and running motions. They did this in order to treat foot disorders they deemed to be caused by biomechanical faults, and, indeed, successful treatments have ensued as a result of the new-found ability to investigate the forces, normal and abnormal, that press on the foot when it is bearing weight. A by-product of this progress is the ability today to deal successfully with foot problems that have been shown to affect parts of the body from the lower back to the ankle. Remember that song about the foot bone being connected to the leg bone, and so on up the body? Well, it is definitely true that problems with foot bones can adversely affect backbones, and all the other bones in between.

Although the study of human biomechanics is still in its relative infancy, it has made rapid strides and, as mentioned, has been particularly enhanced by the recent running/jogging craze. It was the runners with "overuse" syndromes (problems caused by constant normal or abnormal forces on the feet over long periods of time) that convinced previously skeptical medical practitioners that the foot is indeed the culprit in many lower-limb and back ailments. In the four years that I have been podiatric consultant at the Sports Medicine Clinic at the Mount Sinai Hospital in Toronto, my colleagues and I have concluded that over seventy-five per cent of the complaints from the knee down are related directly to poor mechanical function of the lower leg and foot.

The Walking, or Gait, Cycle

It is now time to get down to some basics, and learn what happens when we take a step.

When we speak of the *walking/gait cycle*, we are referring to a person's range of motions when he or she is moving forward. A normal, complete cycle is divided into two separate phases: *stance* and *swing*. The biomechanics of the weight-bearing foot during these phases determine whether or not a person is walking or running normally.

Let us discuss the *stance phase* of the gait cycle first, because it is the most important. The stance phase is divided into three separate parts. The first stage is *contact* and begins at *heel-strike*, that is, the moment when the heel first makes contact with the ground. This represents the first twenty-seven per cent of the stance phase. The second stage is *mid-stance*. It begins with *forefoot-loading*—when the front part of the foot first makes contact with the ground— and ends at *heel-lift*, the point at which the heel is lifting off the ground. Mid-stance represents forty per cent of the stance phase. The final stage of the stance phase is called *propulsive*, and represents thirty-three per cent of that phase. It begins at heel-lift and ends at *toe-off*—when the foot totally leaves the ground and no longer bears any weight. All the parts of the stance phase together account for two-thirds of the total gait, or walking, cycle.

The other third of the gait cycle is the *swing phase*. It is not divided into different components because it occurs when the foot is totally off the ground and not bearing any weight.

The entire gait cycle can be seen in Diagram 3:1.

DIAGRAM 3:1
The Gait Cycle

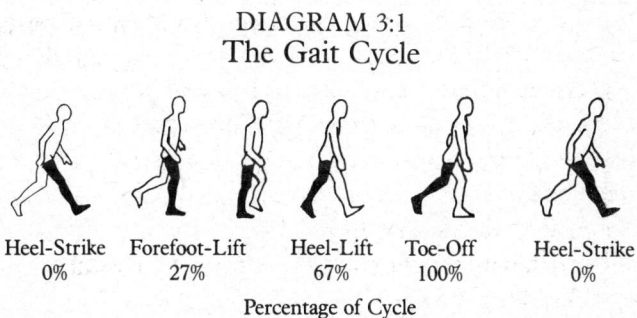

Heel-Strike	Forefoot-Lift	Heel-Lift	Toe-Off	Heel-Strike
0%	27%	67%	100%	0%

Percentage of Cycle

As you may well have understood by now, foot problems develop when something goes wrong during the stance phase of the gait cycle. The basic fault occurs when an abnormal amount of weight is brought to bear on a specific part of the foot; and the primary causes of this abnormal weight-bearing process are biomechanical— more specifically abnormal *pronation* and *supination*.

Pronation and Supination
We shall return shortly to the gait cycle and abnormal biomechan-

ics of the foot. But first it is time to explain the term *supination*, and explain the term *pronation* more fully, because you will be reading a lot about them from now on in this book. Eventually I will be talking about how abnormal pronation and supination can cause foot disorders, but at this point it is important to understand that feet do pronate and supinate a normal amount during the stance phase of the gait cycle. So, when you hear from a person that he or she pronates, or that you pronate, it is an abnormal pronation syndrome that is being referred to.

Pronation involves three distinct motions of the foot during the stance phase (see Diagram 3:2). These motions all occur

DIAGRAM 3:2
Pronation and Supination

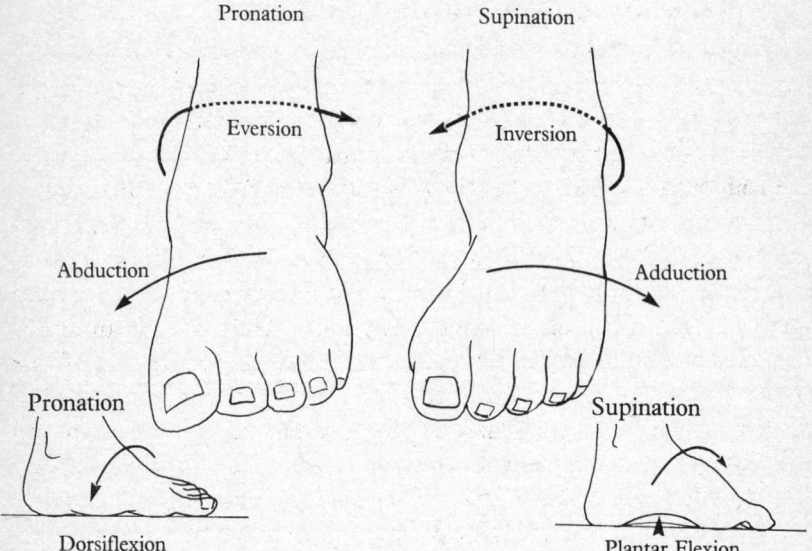

simultaneously and are called *eversion*, *abduction* (not to be confused with kidnapping), and *dorsiflexion*. These words may be Greek to most people, but do not feel discouraged by your lack of knowledge. The average medical student will graduate from medical school and set up practice without ever truly understanding the three terms, or pronation and supination for that matter. Actually, a colleague of mine, who shall remain nameless, still thinks that "pronation" refers to a group of flag-waving patriots.

The foot naturally pronates during the first part (contact) of the stance phase of the gait cycle.

Supination is the exact opposite of pronation, and has absolutely nothing to do with anti-nationalism. The opposing biomechanical movements of the foot are *inversion, adduction,* and *plantar flexion* (see Diagram 3:2). Supination occurs normally during the latter part of the stance phase, from the beginning of the propulsive stage to when the foot lifts off the ground.

Abnormal pronation—the major cause of foot problems—occurs when a foot pronates when it should be supinating, or over-pronates during a normal pronation period of the gait cycle. A foot supinates abnormally when it ought to be pronating, or when it exceeds a normal amount of supination. I will discuss why these abnormalities occur shortly, and throughout the entire book.

As we follow the foot through the gait cycle to find out exactly how much and when the foot pronates and supinates, keep in mind that some amounts of pronation and supination are necessary at certain times to enable the foot to propel forward properly.

From heel-strike almost to the point of forefoot-loading (the contact stage of the stance phase of the gait cycle), the subtalar joint will pronate up to 4° in a normal foot. The joint moves from this pronation to neutral (0°) just after the forefoot hits the ground at mid-stance until the beginning of the propulsive stage. Then it goes from the neutral position to about 4° supination through to the end of the stance phase—at toe-off. At the beginning of the swing phase of the gait cycle, and throughout it, the subtalar joint returns to and remains at about the neutral position. Again, the important thing to remember here is that the foot does normally pronate and supinate during a normal gait cycle, but only up to about 4°. (To remind you of the range of motions of the entire gait cycle, I refer you back to Diagram 3:1.) Another important aspect to remember is that when the foot is neither pronating or supinating, it is in the *neutral* position. A biomechanical problem may exist if the foot is actually pronating or supinating during the stance phase of the gait cycle when it ought to be in the neutral position.

The most crucial joint in the foot affecting the biomechanics of the gait cycle—particularly during the initial stages of the stance phase—is the *subtalar*. You will recall from the last chapter that it comprises three different articulations between the top surface of the heel bone and the bottom surface of the ankle bone.

DIAGRAM 3:3
The Action of the Midtarsal Joints

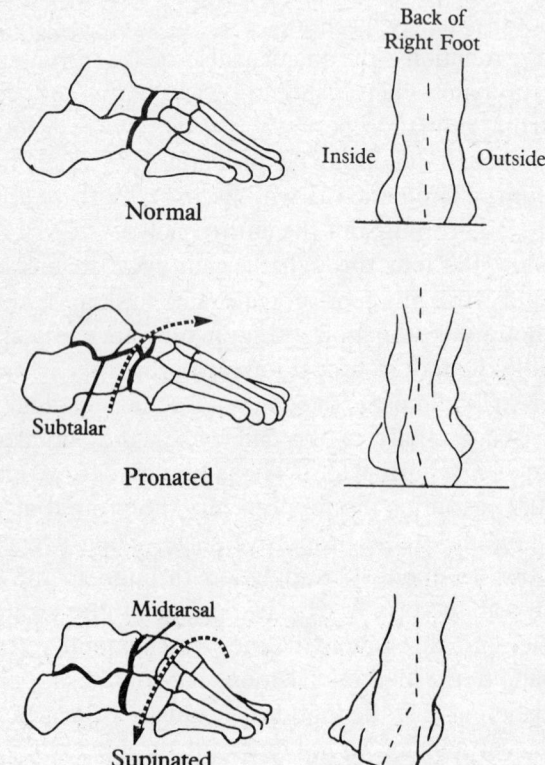

Back of
Right Foot

Normal

Inside   Outside

Subtalar

Pronated

Midtarsal

Supinated

   The subtalar joint works together with the *midtarsal* joint (see Diagram 3:3) to compensate for a temporary pronation or supination problem caused by external factors, such as an uneven terrain, or by a change in upper-body motion—for example, when an athlete kicks a ball or when a ballerina does a pirouette. When these two joints are unable to compensate for a biomechanical problem that is continuous and/or acute, a foot disorder can develop. These disorders will be discussed in detail in the following chapters.

The main stress on the midtarsal joint occurs when the foot is in the mid-stance stage of the stance phase. It becomes more difficult for the midtarsal joint to compensate for a biomechanical problem when the first stage of the stance phase is abnormal and cannot be corrected by the subtalar joint. So, if a person lands abnormally on his or her foot at heel-strike, the possibility exists that the effects of the fault will flow all the way through to the forefoot, where it may manifest itself as some sort of metatarsal-head or toe-joint disorder. The result could be anything from a bunion to a callus or a corn, depending on just where an abnormal amount of weight is being brought to bear on the forefoot.

Abnormal Pronation
Abnormal compensatory pronation is the most common cause of foot disorders. Although there are many reasons why the foot (more specifically the subtalar joint) pronates abnormally, there are five causes, mentioned below, that I see in patients far more than any others. Keep in mind that when a foot has a biomechanical fault there can be an excessive amount of weight focused on a particular part of the foot. It is this overstressing of that part of the foot that causes problems as nature reacts to protect the stressed area, often by forming a layer of protective skin that itself can become irritated, at other times by deviating a bone or soft-tissue mass.

Let me also emphasize here that most of the biomechanical faults causing foot disorders are *congenital* in nature (that is, a person is born with an abnormality, or the propensity to develop one, for whatever reason).

The five most common causes of abnormal pronation are *forefoot varus*, a *plantar-flexed fifth metatarsal head*, *forefoot valgus*, a *rearfoot varus deformity* (see Diagram 3:4), and a lack of motion in the ankle joint. Let me assure the reader that he or she need not be terrified by the medicalese; these conditions are hardly life-threatening, and do not require painful, lengthy treatments to ameliorate. They are simply bony abnormalities that are commonly found to create abnormal pronation.

There are problems in the lower leg that can also cause a foot

DIAGRAM 3:4
Position of the Heel and Toes During Abnormal Pronation

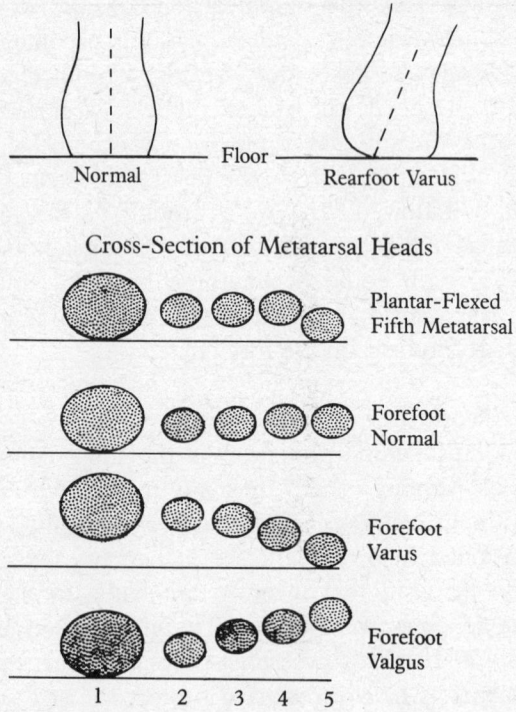

Floor

Normal   Rearfoot Varus

Cross-Section of Metatarsal Heads

Plantar-Flexed
Fifth Metatarsal

Forefoot
Normal

Forefoot
Varus

Forefoot
Valgus

1   2   3   4   5

to pronate abnormally: *tibial varum* (bow legs), *internal tibial* or *femoral torsion*, a short *Achilles tendon* or *calf muscle*, *short hamstring* or *iliopsoas muscles* (see Diagram 3:5), or a discrepancy in lower-limb length. These problems may go unnoticed until a person decides to take up an athletic endeavor. As you will learn in Chapter Fourteen, physical activity will bring to the fore biomechanical faults in the leg and foot that otherwise would not cause any trouble.

As I have mentioned, the reason it is so important to avoid abnormal pronation or supination, is that a biomechanical fault can cause an abnormal amount of force to be focused on one part of the foot. Continuous excessive weight brought to bear on one area of the foot will eventually cause a problem at that site, as you will see in the following chapters. To get an idea of the excessive amounts of weight that are put on a part of the foot when a biomechanical fault exists,

DIAGRAM 3:5
Causes of Pronation

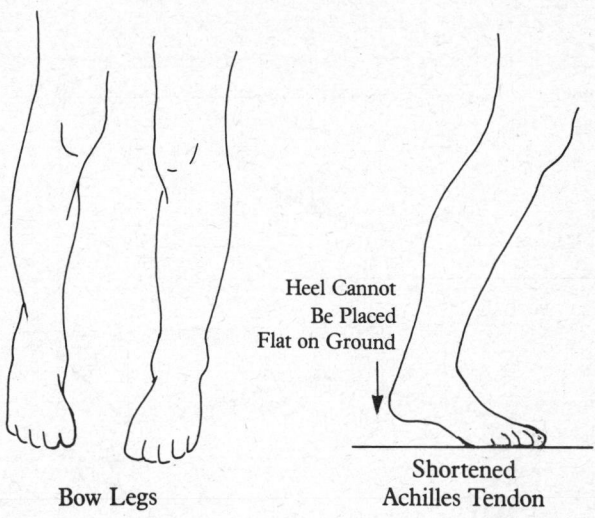

Heel Cannot
Be Placed
Flat on Ground

Bow Legs

Shortened
Achilles Tendon

look at Diagram 3:6, which illustrates how the weight is distributed on the bottom of the foot during normal and abnormal gait cycles.

Abnormal Supination

Supination will receive short shrift in this book, and the reason is that abnormal supination accounts for a small percentage of all the foot problems I have seen in my years as a podiatrist. I am sure that my practice is no different from that of my podiatrist colleagues throughout North America. The typical supinating foot is one with a high arch and rigid structure (see Diagram 3:7). There may often be a neuro-muscular component to the problem causing the supination syndrome.

Examining for a Biomechanical Foot Fault

Once a foot specialist has learned the tricks of the trade, his/her trained eye can make many precise judgments. So it is when examining a patient for a biomechanical problem. I can judge the relationships between the foot and the leg of a patient by watching him or her walk barefoot on a flat surface. I can tell whether they are pronating

DIAGRAM 3:6
Pressure Areas on the Sole of the Foot During Normal and Pronated Gait

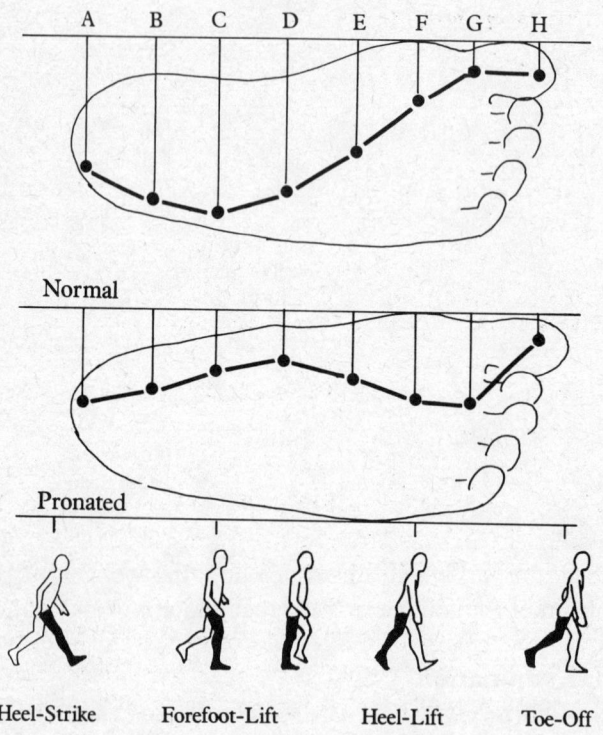

Normal

Pronated

Heel-Strike   Forefoot-Lift   Heel-Lift   Toe-Off

or supinating abnormally, or if they have any other biomechanical fault.

Also, while no two feet are alike, there are those far enough from the norm that their idiosyncrasies can be spotted by the experienced naked eye. The two most common features of an abnormally shaped foot are the high arch (*pes cavus*), which is somewhat rigid, and the low arch (*pes planus*) (see Diagram 3:7).

The high-arched foot is often, but not always, somewhat rigid, and it is a poorer shock-absorber than the normal arch. Its shape exposes the metatarsal heads (the ends of the metatarsal bones that articulate with the toe bones) of the foot to added pressure when the forefoot is bearing weight. As a result, numerous forefoot disorders can arise, although there are many people with high-arched

DIAGRAM 3:7
Two Biomechanical Faults of the Foot

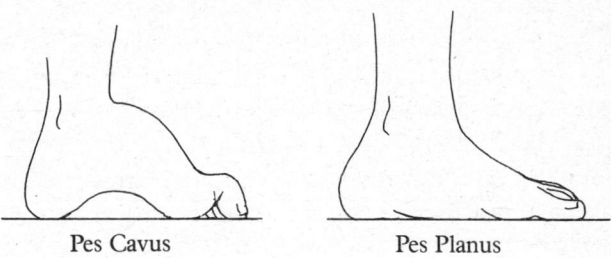

Pes Cavus   Pes Planus

feet who are fine unless they take up some activity or wear certain shoes that may put even more stress on the forefoot during the walking cycle.

The Myth of Flat Feet and Fallen Arches
I will try my best to avoid corny jokes about flat feet and fallen arches. Suffice it to say that biomechanical problems of the feet have been discussed by the medical profession for at least fifty years, and so-called flat feet have been used as an excuse by artful draft-dodgers in various wars to avoid military service. Thus there have been a lot of stories told about these conditions for at least a half-century. Also, there are numerous anecdotes and jokes about flatfoots—policemen who have walked the beat for too long—and dim-witted or slow-moving individuals who have been caught flat-footed. So, despite attempts by the medical profession—or, perhaps, with its help on occasion—the flat foot and the fallen arch have become widely accepted myths, much like the slipped disc. But feet are rarely flat, and arches do not fall; they only seem that way because of poor biomechanics of the foot.

True flat feet are basically congenital, and they are rarely seen. But the low-arched foot is not necessarily abnormal, and it is definitely not *flat*. However, the shape of the foot makes it conducive to over-pronation during the gait cycle, and, as a result, it appears flat when weight is brought to bear on it.

Although I can diagnose a biomechanical fault, such as a patient's over-pronation, with my naked eye, I am not a computer or some other space-age diagnostic tool. Therefore, I cannot measure precisely the exact amount of pronation in a foot at a given point of the gait cycle. However, there is new diagnostic equipment on the market today that we hope will revolutionize the examination of the gait cycle of a patient so that adjustments, in the form of an insert that is fitted into the shoe, can be made to correct a fault.

I will again be discussing these inserts (*orthotics*) later in the chapter. At this point, though, I would like to caution the reader that orthotics are not always miracle-workers, although the success rate with their use is high.

An Example of a Biomechanical Fault Causing a Foot Disorder

I hope that you now understand the fundamentals of the biomechanics of the motions of the foot as it goes through the walking cycle. In a sense, motion flows down through the leg, through the ankle and the subtalar joint, through the midtarsal joint, and all the way down to and across the metatarsal heads to the big, or great, toe. I also trust that you can see why a biomechanical fault can lead to a foot disorder: by causing an abnormal amount of weight to be focused on one part of the foot. Let me now illustrate how the biomechanical fault can occur, usually as a result of a congenital foot abnormality, and how it can affect a person from the foot all the way up to the lower back. Keep in mind that I am able to diagnose the problem by watching the patient walk and by examining the foot. In certain cases I will also be able to pinpoint the degree of the biomechanical fault by using modern diagnostic equipment that has recently become available to medical practitioners.

In the abnormal foot, the toes of which are shown in cross-section in Diagram 3:8, the second metatarsal bone (the second-largest bone in the forefoot) is closer to the ground than the other four metatarsal bones. As a result, more pressure is being applied to that bone during the latter part of the stance phase of the gait cycle than to other metatarsal bones. Because that bone bears excessive weight owing to its abnormal positioning, the bottom of the bone will eventually become inflamed. This sets off a chain reaction. A callus will form on the skin under the bone, causing it to become even

DIAGRAM 3:8
Formation of a Callus Under a Plantar-Flexed Metatarsal Head

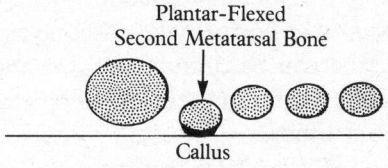

Plantar-Flexed
Second Metatarsal Bone

Callus

Cross-Section of
Metatarsal Heads

more inflamed and bruised from the pounding it is receiving, and from the stress of the callus.

Eventually the pain will become severe enough in the area that the victim will try to compensate by shifting his/her weight to the baby-toe side of the foot, thereby creating an abnormal supination syndrome. This imbalanced, abnormal walking or running gait will affect the biomechanics of the entire foot and leg, and can create discomfort on the outside of the knee and in the hip. This is because all the muscles and tendons in those areas are being over-extended, and the knee and hip joints are, therefore, becoming inflamed.

Once the original problem—the abnormally positioned second metatarsal bone—is treated, the biomechanics of the lower extremities should normalize, and, if the conditions have not been allowed to go on for too long, all the symptoms will disappear.

The above example illustrates the "Leaning Tower of Pisa Syndrome" that I mentioned earlier, and shows how a foot problem can adversely affect other parts of the body. Of course, this syndrome can operate in reverse. An abnormal calf muscle can place added strain on the Achilles tendon, and subsequently on the ankle joint. This could create a pronation problem in the subtalar joint and, therefore, a biomechanical fault that did not begin in the foot. As a result, added pressure may be put on a part of the foot when it is bearing weight, and an inflammation could develop.

Arthritis
The Leaning Tower of Pisa Syndrome often leads to an arthritic condition—specifically to *osteoarthritis*.

I would like to remind you here that, in my opinion, osteoarthritis is not a disease. This is a belief that I share with many of my orthopedic colleagues. A simple wear-and-tear process in any body joint can precipitate an inflammation, because of the breakdown of the cartilage tissue that normally keeps bone from rubbing against bone. Cartilage tissue can be unduly stressed and broken down by abnormal forces in the joint, forces that often result from a biomechanical fault in the lower limbs.

If an athlete or a dancer regularly places excessive stress on the lower limbs while performing or exercising, the joints in the lower extremities of the body will be subjected to more wear-and-tear than the joints of people who do not partake in overly strenuous activity. No disease is actually destroying any of the stressed joints; normal, external, but excessive biomechanical forces are causing the condition. Would you expect even the best tires on a racing car to last forever? Even on a normal car, an excellent set of tires will have to be replaced after fifty to seventy-five thousand miles. But the tires are neither diseased nor faulty, just worn down. The same applies to the joints in our bodies. However, we often help speed up the degeneration process by allowing a biomechanical fault or excessive stress to continue until a joint has been sufficiently inflamed to cause discomfort and, eventually, dysfunction.

When you allow a biomechanical fault to continue untreated, you are helping along the wear-and-tear process in the joints in your feet, legs, hips, and lower back, because you are constantly placing undue stress on those joints in order to walk or run.

In actual practice, about ninety per cent of all common foot pain, including osteoarthritis, is caused by abnormal biomechanical forces. And, just as faulty wheel-alignment in a car can result in tire wear-and-tear, the abnormal forces due to misalignment in your lower limbs can cause early wear-and-tear in the joints in your feet. As we have already discussed, foot problems can create havoc in the entire bottom half of your body. However, with proper mechanical adjustments—for example, the wearing of *orthotics*—further wear-and-tear can be prevented, and pain can be drastically reduced, or even eliminated altogether in many cases.

If you look at Diagram 3:9, you will see examples of how poor biomechanics of the foot can throw out the alignment of your body

DIAGRAM 3:9
Effects of Lower-Body Alignment on Biomechanics

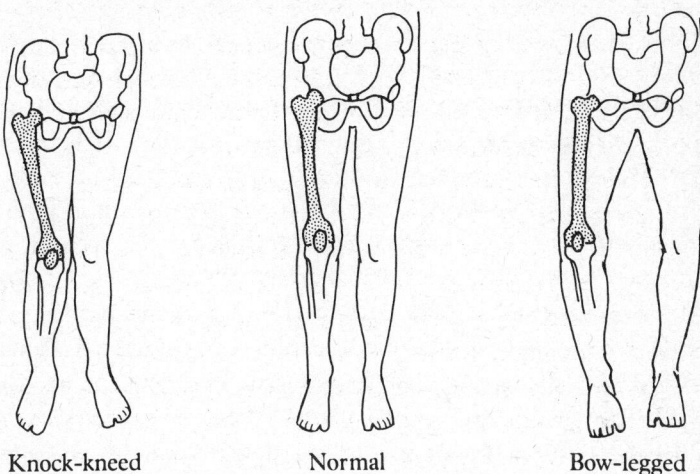

Knock-kneed   Normal   Bow-legged

from the lower back down, and cause excessive stress on certain joints.

There are other forms of arthritis—*rheumatoid*, *gouty*, and *psoriatic*, to name the most common of them—that are called *systemic arthritic diseases*. They are caused by internal disorders that can be classified as diseases rather than as non-disease wear-and-tear, and they too can result in severe damage to the joints. However, these diseases are much rarer than osteoarthritis. In fact, fewer than a half of one per cent of my "arthritic" patients suffer from the systemic-disease varieties. I will discuss the more common of these diseases in Chapter Eleven.

Orthotics
The last thing I want to talk about in this chapter is the *orthotic* device that fits into a shoe, and is designed to properly redistribute the weight on the foot and correct any abnormal foot motions.

In the past fifteen years there has been tremendous progress in the research and development of sophisticated shoe inserts that are made from special materials and are molded to eliminate abnormal weight-bearing forces on the foot. In some cases, a biomechanical fault can be treated by a simple over-the-counter insert, but many people require a device molded specifically for their foot. These devices cannot be purchased over the counter, although many people believe that they are indeed purchasing "orthotics" in stores that sell foot-care and footwear products. What many of them are actually buying is an "arch support" that is quite different from an orthotic device.

An orthotic device is generally considered to be a custom-made shoe insert, designed specifically for a particular foot. It is intended to properly redistribute the weight on the bottom of the foot, and it aids in correcting abnormal foot motion. The least important task of a true orthotic device is supporting the arch. However, arch supports do aid in preventing mild abnormal pronation, and in cases where a simple arch support is indicated, it should be considered instead of a much more expensive orthotic. I would, though, draw the analogy of a magnifying glass and a state-of-the-art contact lens or pair of glasses. If you need only to read small print, a magnifying glass will suffice if your eyes are otherwise normal; but if you have a specific vision impairment, such as an astigmatism, you will need properly customized glasses or contact lenses.

For those people who require sophisticated orthotics that are molded specially for their feet, the procedure is simple and fairly quick, if a bit messy. A mold is made from a plaster cast of the foot of the patient. That mold is then sent to a special laboratory, where the orthotic inserts are designed from the shape of the plaster cast.

I want to caution again that orthotics are not always miracle-workers, although the success rate with their use is quite high. I have had a few disappointed patients come back to me with no relief from their problem after wearing specially designed orthotic devices for a prescribed period of time. At that point I have to inform these patients that other modes of treatment may be advisable. I will discuss the use of orthotics in great detail as they pertain to specific bio-mechanical disorders in subsequent chapters. And I will explain why they do not always work.

4

The Bunion, and Other Big-Toe Abnormalities

As I was preparing this chapter, a medical colleague of mine informed me with a straight face that he intended to specialize in the near future on stomach surgery and podiatry so that he could enjoy his favourite dish—chopped liver and bunions.

I suspect that bunion sufferers will not find the humor to their taste, because the removal of a painful bunion is not a simple matter, although modern surgical techniques have certainly reduced trauma to the patient and enhanced the chances of a successful outcome.

A Historical Perspective of the Bunion

The word *bunion* may actually have been derived from the old English word "bunny", which meant "a small swelling". But the history of the bunion goes back much farther than that.

Man has been plagued and intrigued for centuries by bunions. If you were to examine closely some of the earliest Egyptian drawings and writings, you would see and find descriptions of feet obviously deformed by bunions and other big-toe abnormalities. However, it appears that foot surgeons began experimenting with various surgical techniques only in the 1800s, and rarely with great success. One of the problems was that they adapted procedures from common types of hand surgery. Unfortunately, people do not normally stand or walk on their hands. The hand is not a weight-bearing appendage, unlike the foot, so operations that failed to take into consideration the fact that man constantly puts weight on his feet failed miserably. Also, in those days, disinfection of the instruments, the surgeon's hands, the patient's feet, and the bandaging was not a priority.

Therefore, many patients who had foot surgery developed severe complications post-operatively.

Tall Bunion Tales

Contrary to some fairy tales, a bunion is not a skin disorder; neither is it commonly caused by ill-fitting shoes, although shoes can precipitate the condition in some cases. It annoys me that a popular medical dictionary states that bunions "are usually caused by ill-fitting shoes." Why then do certain people living in tropical climes, who have never worn shoes, suffer continuously from bunions? Many people also believe that once they have a bunion, they are stuck with it for life. They believe that the only possible way to rid themselves of the abnormality is to undergo painful surgery, and a lengthy and uncomfortable recuperation period. As you will learn in this chapter, many bunions can be treated without surgical intervention, and, fortunately, the surgical horror stories of the past century are ancient history. Bunion surgery today is quite sophisticated and relatively painless, and the recuperation period takes much less time than you might have imagined.

Why Bunions Develop

A bunion (in medicalese, *hallux valgus*) literally defined is *hallux* (big, or great, toe) and *valgus* (deforming away from the midline). What it means in plain English is that there is a deviation in the big-toe joint, and in Diagram 4:1 you can see how an abnormal big toe deviates from the shape of a normal big toe. Strictly speaking, however, a bunion is a bump, while a hallux valgus is a deviation of the big toe, so the two terms are not identical in meaning. But, since they are normally synonymous, I have chosen to use the terms interchangeably, and I hope my purist colleagues will forgive me.

Extensive research into the cause and prevention of bunions was enhanced by the frustrating realization over the past few decades that bunions often recur after surgical treatment. Eventually it was discovered that almost all people with bunions pronated abnormally. Using early medical knowledge and theories of cause and effect, researchers initially deduced that bunions caused abnormal pronation. In other words, a bunion could adversely affect the biomechanics of the foot. However, the researchers quickly realized that this was akin to saying that tension relieved sex, and that the reverse was true: pronation caused bunions.

I am forever being questioned by patients about the heredity factor of bunions. If your grandmother and mother had bunions, will you also succumb to the disorder? The answer is that, while a hereditary predisposition may exist, the bunions can be prevented if the causes are eliminated. The shape of a person's foot is obviously determined to a great extent by genetics, just like the color of one's hair, eyes, and skin, so a person may be born with a foot that is susceptible to abnormal pronation. However, with proper foot care from the beginning, the incidence of inherited bunions can be dramatically reduced, even eliminated.

I listed the major causes of abnormal pronation in the last chapter. The majority of cases involving bunions actually involve two bio-mechanical faults—a combination of abnormal subtalar joint pronation and a foot that has an excessively flexible first metatar-sal bone. When these two conditions exist, the big-toe joint will be called upon to absorb a tremendous amount of weight when the foot is about to push off the ground at the end of the stance phase of the gait cycle—the push-off at the end of the propulsive stage.

DIAGRAM 4:1
Formation of a Bunion

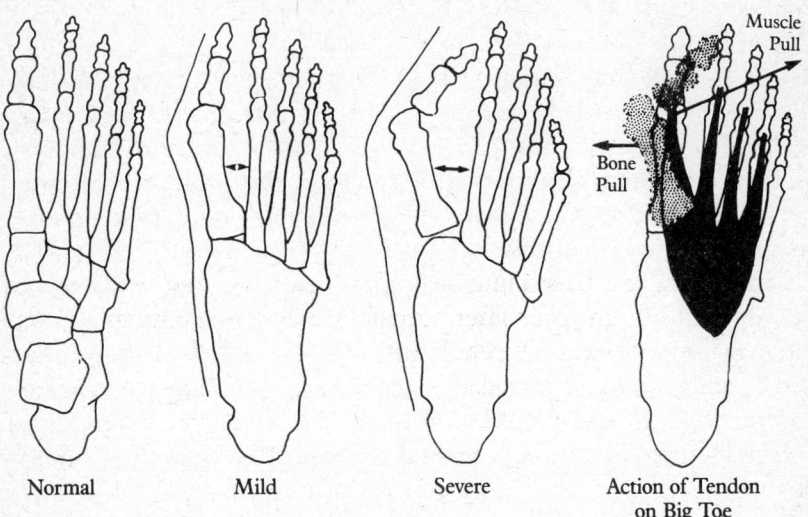

| Normal | Mild | Severe | Action of Tendon on Big Toe |

The reason is that the tendons in the big toe are being asked to stretch and function in a radically elongated position as they try to counteract the abnormal forces of the pronation and the overly flexible first metatarsal bone. This action of the tendons places enormous tension on the big toe, eventually forcing it to deviate to the outside with the top of the toe pointing towards the baby toe (also Diagram 4:1). This situation results in the big toe exerting pressure on the first metatarsal bone, which is subsequently pulled to the outside. So, the *proximal phalanx* (the big bone in the big toe) and the first metatarsal bone are being pulled in opposite directions—like a wishbone. What a person with a bunion winds up with is often a grotesquely shaped toe as a result of opposing forces that do not counterbalance each other without causing a deformity.

Diagnosing a bunion is not difficult for a foot specialist. If you examine a weight-bearing foot and find a bump at the big-toe joint where there ought not to be one, you are looking at a bunion.

There are three basic types of bunion: mild, moderate, and severe. The terminology has nothing to do with the amount of pain involved or the degree of cartilage wear-and-tear in the big-toe joint. It refers specifically to the actual degree of deviation of the joint. There are other big-toe joint disorders that involve almost no deformity but produce much more pain than even a severe bunion.

Treating the Bunion
When it comes to treating a bunion, it is logical to assume that the milder the case, the less involved the treatment. In fact, mild, painless bunions that cause no significant discomfort or dysfunction ought to be treated conservatively, basically by the fitting of an orthotic device to eliminate the over-pronation of the foot, and thus to prevent further deviation of the big-toe joint.

Since bunions do involve the big-toe joint, and since the joints of the body can become inflamed from irritation (for example, from wearing overly tight shoes) and, as a result, can become painful, it may occasionally be necessary to treat a mild, but irritated, bunion with an anti-inflammatory drug for a short period of time. There are two types of anti-inflammatories available: *steroid* and *nonsteroidal*. Steroid drugs belong to the *cortisone* family and are often quite effective. But they carry with them potentially harmful side effects. Non-steroidal drugs are also effective when used for the right reasons, but they also carry with them side effects—especially to the gastro-intestinal tract, in the form of irritation, and possible ulceration and bleeding.

I will have more to say about anti-inflammatory drugs in subsequent chapters, but I would like to point out here that I use them with great discretion, and only to relieve an inflammation, not to cure a particular condition. My main concern with anti-inflammatory drugs, aside from the potentially harmful side effects, is that they do not treat the underlying causes of most of the disorders with which I come in contact. As I stated earlier, most of the patients I see have biomechanical faults that will continue to cause discomfort until they have been successfully dealt with. Neither abnormal pronation nor a bunion can be eliminated by an anti-inflammatory drug, which only partially controls the inflammatory process.

Cortisone injections fall into the same category as anti-inflammatory medications taken orally. Although they can be quite successful in the treatment of severe joint pain, the benefits do not always outweigh the overall risks that may occur with the injection of a steroid into a joint. Many medical experts strongly believe that cortisone injections into any joint, including the big-toe joint, can accelerate deterioration of the cartilage in that area, thereby negating in the long run any short-term pain relief. It is generally left to the discretion of the physician, after consultation with the patient and evaluation of the risks and benefits presented by the injection of the steroid, to determine whether or not to proceed with the cortisone treatment. To repeat, however, as far as I am concerned, the original biomechanical fault causing the inflammation must be dealt with in order to negate the need for such anti-inflammatory medication.

Physiotherapy is another possibility in the treatment of a mild bunion that is painful. Whirlpool baths and ultrasound may help relieve the inflammation and thereby speed up the healing process in the area. Manipulation therapy may also help at times; it is usually a pleasant experience to be massaged or rubbed, particularly where there is discomfort. Manipulation can aid the restoration of a normal range of motion in the big-toe joint, but it will not eliminate the abnormal pronation causing the problem. So, physiotherapy, like other modes of treatment, will fail in the long run because the bio-mechanical fault has yet to be overcome.

Aligning the Toe

Unfortunately, many of my bunion patients seek help when they are already past the stage of conservative treatment. For them the options are generally limited to surgery or to walking barefoot—or in grossly oversized shoes—for the rest of their lives.

Over the past fifteen or so years there have been tremendous strides in the surgical removal of bunions. Previously, there were basically two or three procedures in a surgeon's repertoire for bunion correction. Usually patients were hospitalized, operated on under a general anesthetic, kept in the hospital for seven to ten days, and placed in a non-walking cast for four to eight weeks. Today almost all bunion surgery can be performed on an out-patient basis, even in a doctor's office, and under a local anesthetic. A non-walking cast is not required, and the patient can convalesce quite comfortably at home. Recovery time will vary with the severity of the condition, but it is normally much faster than with the old surgical techniques. The surgery can be performed by either an orthopedic specialist or a podiatrist. Although the orthopedic surgeon specializing in feet may use a slightly different technique from the podiatrist, the results ought to be the same. I would not hesitate to recommend any number of surgeons from both fields.

Most foot surgeons are trained to use either *open* or *closed* (minimal-incision) surgery techniques; usually the method is determined by the nature of the case. At present, both procedures play an important role, but I expect that in the near future foot surgeons will be operating on bunions using new techniques that incorporate the best of both worlds.

In "open" bunion surgery, a two- to four-inch incision is made to expose the area to be operated on. Once the incision has been completed, the deformity can be repaired by redesigning the offending bone with new power equipment.

"Closed" minimal-incision surgery (M.I.S.) is done through a *stab* incision no more than ⅛" wide (Diagram 4:2). A small *burr* (a type of drill) is introduced through the incision and deep into the tissue. Surgery is performed by touch and feel. The surgeon does not actually see the offending bone structure, so in a sense he is "flying blind".

DIAGRAM 4:2
Surgical Techniques (shown during bunion surgery)

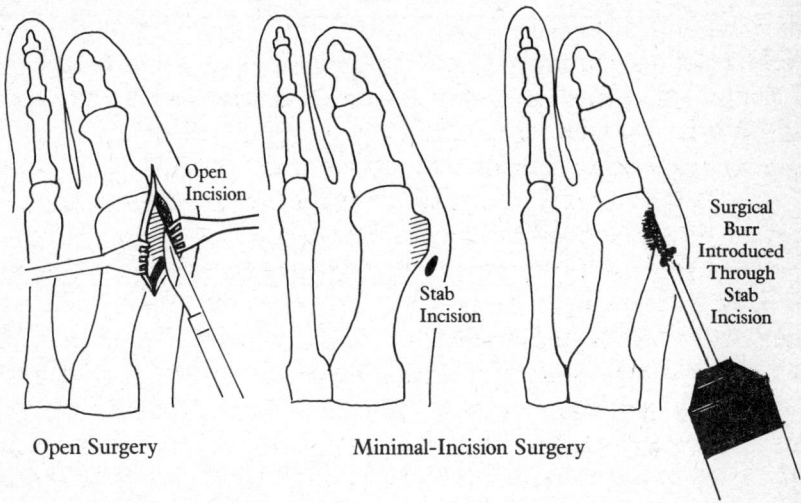

Open
Incision

Surgical
Burr
Introduced
Through
Stab
Incision

Stab
Incision

Open Surgery   Minimal-Incision Surgery

This technique demands not only a much greater "feel" by the surgeon, but an explicit understanding of the anatomy of the area. According to "closed" surgeons, the benefits of M.I.S. are: less tissue destruction than with open surgery, less trauma to the bone, and less chance of infection.

On the other hand, those who favor "open" surgery techniques argue that there is less chance of error when the area to be operated on is totally exposed. Also, they believe that the use of the burr can be even more traumatic to soft tissue around the bone than is a sharp scalpel.

It is my opinion that M.I.S. has helped revolutionize foot care. However, there may have been a tendency in podiatry in the last ten years to proclaim it as the be-all and end-all in foot surgery. There is indeed much controversy in medical circles today as to the pros and cons of M.I.S. Some experts have gone so far as to call M.I.S. a gimmick. I believe that, with further advances, M.I.S. on the foot will become more accepted. But I also feel that there will always be conditions that will require more conventional "open" procedures.

Before deciding on the bunion-surgery technique, it is imperative to determine the shape and position of the large big-toe joint. As you can plainly see from Diagram 4:3, the big-toe bone (proximal phalanx) in a normal foot sits directly ahead of the first metatarsal bone, and lies in an almost straight line when the foot is not in motion. The cartilage of the joint is in a healthy condition and the big toe has a range of motion, moving up or down, of at least forty-five degrees. This is not the case with a deformed big-toe joint.

DIAGRAM 4:3
A Normal and a Fused Big-Toe Joint

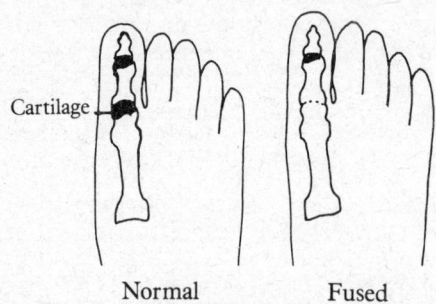

Cartilage

Normal   Fused

The two major concerns with bunions are: (a) the position of the metatarsal head vis-à-vis the big-toe joint, and (b) the condition of the cartilage in the joint. Often when a forefoot deformity exists, an actual bunion does not form in the big toe. But there is so much wear-and-tear on the big-toe joint that the cartilage erodes, and the joint surface flattens. As a result, the range of motion of the big-toe joint diminishes. When this happens, the condition is called *hallux limitus*. Hallux limitus does not refer to a celestial body, it simply means "limited motion of the big toe". In severe cases, where no motion exists at all in the big-toe joint, *hallux rigidus* occurs. As you have probably guessed, this condition is a totally rigid big-toe joint.

In some cases, as you can see on the right in Diagram 4:3, when the cartilage has totally worn out and the joint between the first metatarsal bone and the big-toe bone has become perfectly rigid, the two bones become fused and the joint itself ceases to exist. What exists instead is one long bone, so, while the area now becomes pain-free, there can no longer be any normal joint motion. As a result, the person with such a condition loses a lot of physical mobility.

It is only after the surgeon has fully evaluated the condition of the big-toe joint by the use of X-rays and manipulation of the toe that he can determine precisely which of the techniques in his repertoire best suit the situation. A badly damaged joint will obviously require a totally different approach from that used to treat a mild bunion and a relatively unaffected joint. And, as I have already mentioned, it is entirely possible to have big-toe-joint damage, with little or no cartilage remaining, but not have a bunion. In that case, the surgical procedure changes again.

Hallux Limitus and Hallux Rigidus
As I mentioned above, these two conditions may or may not accompany bunions, and they may be much more painful. They can respond well to anti-inflammatory medication, physiotherapy, or orthotic devices, but surgical intervention may be required if the discomfort and dysfunction caused by these conditions become unbearable for the patient.

You recall that hallux limitus refers to restricted, usually painful, motion of the big-toe joint. On the other hand, a person suffering from hallux rigidus has almost no motion in the big-toe joint and can experience a great deal of pain until it fuses. These conditions are illustrated in Diagram 4:4.

DIAGRAM 4:4
Conditions Which Restrict Big-Toe-Joint Movement

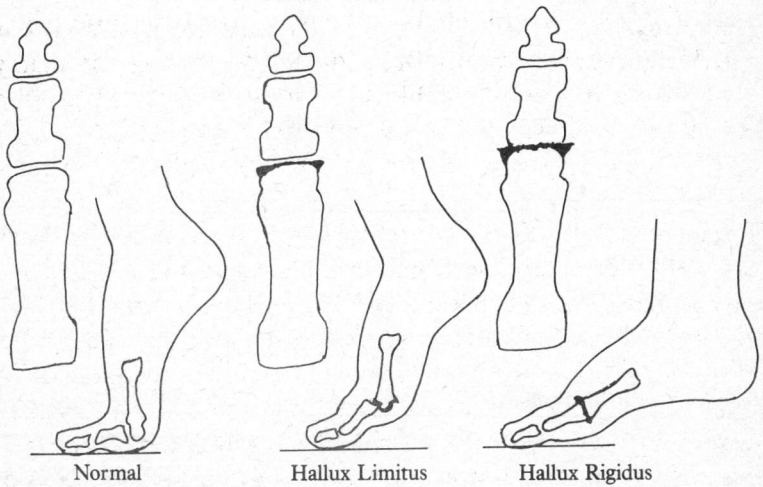

Normal   Hallux Limitus   Hallux Rigidus

Hallux limitus and hallux rigidus are wear-and-tear arthritic disorders (osteoarthritis), not diseases. They are examples of painful manifestations of a biomechanical fault. As usual, the culprit is probably abnormal pronation that results in excess weight being brought to bear on the big-toe joint—weight that the joint was not designed to accept easily. The actual pain in the big-toe joint is caused by the wear-and-tear process that acts to destroy the cushioning cartilage at the ends of the bones. As a result, bone begins to rub against bone—in this case the head of the metatarsal bone and the end of the big-toe bone—and the irritation produces an inflammation that causes pain. The situation could be compared to throwing sand into a ball-bearing joint in a piece of machinery. The machinery cannot run smoothly with the foreign objects grinding on its moving parts. This pain in the big-toe joint is often mistaken for *gout*, or some other systemic arthritic-type disease. But, in ninety-nine per cent of the cases, the problem is osteoarthritis, which, as you know, is not a disease at all. It pains me that I see at least one patient each week who is being treated by medication for gout, even though all the blood tests for the disease were negative. I shall have much more to say about gout in Chapter Eleven. Although it affects the big-toe joint, it belongs in a discussion of systemic diseases that affect the foot.

It is possible to treat hallux limitus and hallux rigidus non-surgically, as we would treat a mild bunion, if the diagnosis is made early enough, before severe deterioration of the joint has taken place. However, if deterioration of the joint is extensive and the pain is severe, surgical intervention must be considered, particularly for hallux rigidus. There are three quite successful open-surgery procedures that all involve repair of the big-toe joint.

Post-operative Care
Just because bunion and other big-toe surgery no longer has to be done in a hospital, the patient must not be lulled into believing that the toe will miraculously recover all by itself. There are numerous rules for the patient to follow. Since the recovery routines will vary with the severity of the operation, I will not attempt to go into great detail here about what to do and what not to do. What I do want to stress here, and throughout the book, is the necessity for the

patient to communicate with the surgeon, and to understand fully what he or she must do following surgery to ensure a rapid, trouble-free recovery. As you might suspect, the more involved the surgery, the lengthier the recuperation period. In any event you will not be able to run a marathon immediately following the operation. On the other hand, if you follow the surgeon's instructions, you should be relatively free of discomfort post-operatively, and you ought to be able to resume normal physical activities in a matter of weeks.

A Final Word Before Leaving the Joint

I hate to continuously belabor the point, but I must re-emphasize my belief that, regardless of the condition of the big toe and the need for surgery, the biomechanical fault causing a big-toe problem must be eliminated with a proper orthotic device to prevent the renewed deterioration and/or deviation of the big-toe joint. Otherwise, no matter how much you play around with the big-toe joint, the problems will continue. The sole exception to this caveat is when the cause of the trouble is a systemic disorder. I will discuss the treatment of such conditions in Chapter Eleven.

I must also reiterate my plea for the need for a patient and a doctor to fully understand each other. A patient must know precisely what bunion or other big-toe surgery will do for him or her, and the doctor must be aware of the expectations of the patient. A patient who does not get what he or she bargained for will not be happy. As an example, the following fictional conversation between patient and surgeon quite fairly illustrates the type of misinformation that is often received in a doctor's office by both parties.

PATIENT: Doc, my big toe really hurts.

DOCTOR: Well, it's no wonder. The X-rays indicate substantial arthritis in the joint. (What he means is that the patient has hallux rigidus. However, he does not describe the condition in detail because he does not believe that the patient will understand. He does suspect, however, that the patient will know something about arthritis.) We may have to operate.

PATIENT: Geez, Doc, arthritis . . . an operation. Can you fix me up so that I don't have to miss too much work? Will the pain go away?

DOCTOR: Don't worry. I'll simply remove the joint, using a new procedure, and the pain will be gone for good. You'll be back to work in no time.

PATIENT: That's great, Doc. When can I get it over with?

The patient has heard that his arthritis will be totally relieved. Although the doctor has not said so, the patient also believes that his big toe will be perfectly normal again. The patient fails to ask about potential side effects of the surgery. Either he does not suspect that there will be any, or he does not want to know, as long as the pain is eliminated. The doctor either forgets to tell the patient about the side effects of the operation, which involves fusion of the big-toe joint, or decides that the patient will not understand or will not want to know for whatever reason. As a result, the patient winds up with a painless, fused big toe that he cannot manipulate, rather than the painless big toe with a normal range of motion that he expected. He has unwittingly sacrificed a degree of mobility for pain relief, and he feels that the operation was less than totally successful. On the other hand, the surgeon believes that the operation was a total success, since it accomplished precisely what it set out to do: eliminate the patient's pain completely.

The moral of this story is: If you are the patient, do not hesitate to ask all the questions that come into your mind; if you are the doctor, make sure that the patient fully understands the nature of the condition, the treatment involved, and the potential side effects of that treatment. This communication will save both sides a lot of misery.

The Bunionette

Finally, it was brought to my attention by one of my medical colleagues who was reading over this chapter that I had forgotten to mention the *bunionette*. There is good reason for this apparent oversight. The bunionette, also known as a *baby bunion* or a *tailor's bunion*, occurs on the fifth, or baby toe. Therefore I wish to deal with it in detail in Chapter Six, which discusses forefoot abnormalities, rather than in this chapter, which has focused on the big toe.

5
Hammer Toes and Corns

I am not introducing a new detective series in this chapter. Hammer toes and corns are conditions that affect the foot—and they often go together. I will explain to you shortly why that is so, but first let me tell you a little about the corn, because I know many of you are quite curious, and often misinformed, about them.

A Kernel of Truth
The word "corn", as it applies to a protrusion on the skin, has absolutely nothing to do with the plant that sprouts ears. It comes from the Latin word *cornu*, which means literally "horn". Obviously, somewhere and at some time during the course of European history, the comparison was made between the thickened area of skin that arises on or between toes and a horny protuberance. Hence the English word "corn".

In medicalese, a corn is called a *heloma*, and by definition it is a protrusion on the top or the side of a toe. About two-thirds of all corns occur on the top of the toe and develop in response to contraction of the offending toe. The toe has been bent because of a biomechanical foot-fault, or, occasionally, because of the wearing of improperly fitting shoes. A third of all corns are so-called "soft" or "wet" corns, and occur on the sides of the toes. These are also caused primarily by a biomechanical fault.

Some people confuse corns and *calluses*. The difference between the two is that the callus appears only on the bottom of the foot. However, both are thickened areas of skin, and both are caused primarily by biomechanical foot faults. We will discuss calluses in

57

the next chapter, but if you look at Diagram 5:1, you will see what a typical callus and a typical corn look like, and where one of them may develop on the foot.

DIAGRAM 5:1
Sites of Corns and Calluses

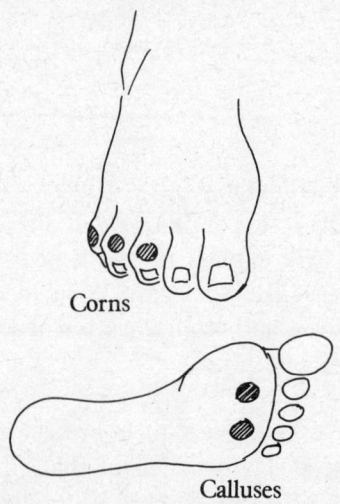

Corns

Calluses

I will discuss "soft" corns later in the chapter, but first I want to talk about those corns that form on top of the toes, and about what usually causes them—hammer toes.

The Hammered Toe

One of the primary causes of corns on the top of the toe is the *hammer toe*, which is not a device for banging nails into the floor. As you can see in Diagram 5:2, a hammer toe is unusually contracted and bent. This situation develops over a period of years, and finally reaches the point at which it becomes obvious and painful. Unfortunately, a person will not normally notice its development until the area begins to hurt, and by then fitting into a pair of shoes can be a very painful experience.

Speaking of shoes, the common belief is that tight and other poorly fitting shoes are the primary causes of hammer toes. I beg to differ. One has only to examine the feet of African Bushmen, who have never worn any shoes, to discover that many of them also suffer from hammer toes.

So, if shoes are not normally to blame for the development of hammer toes, what is? As you may have suspected, the culprit is generally our old friend the biomechanical fault. But this time we have to look at the muscles and tendons on top of and below the toe bones to discover how they can cause the toe to form into the shape of a hammer. If you examine Diagram 5:2, you will be able to see exactly where these muscles and tendons are situated.

DIAGRAM 5:2
A Hammer Toe and the Extensor and Flexor Tendons

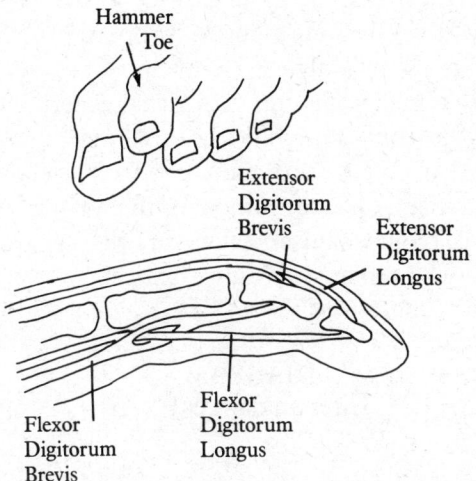

We are going to talk here about *flexor* and *extensor* muscles, so allow me to explain briefly the difference between the two. Flexor muscles cause bending movements of a limb or other body part; extensor muscles, on the other hand, cause a straightening movement.

The muscles on top of all the toes, with the exception of the big toe, are called the *extensor digitorum longus* and the *extensor digitorum brevis*. Those on the underside of the four toes are called the *flexor digitorum longus* and the *flexor digitorum brevis*. The corresponding muscles on the big toe are the *extensor hallucis longus*, the *extensor hallucis brevis*, the *flexor hallucis longus*, and the *flexor hallucis brevis.* Together these muscles control the movements of the toe. When something happens, for whatever reason, to cause at least one of the muscles to malfunction, the biomechanics of the toe involved will also become abnormal. The most common result will be a hammer toe. Once a hammer toe exists, a corn cannot be far behind.

Incidentally, all the toes with the exception of the big toe have three bones, so there are two *interphalangeal joints* in each of the four lesser toes (see Diagram 5:3). When we refer to hammer toes, we mean a *contracture* of the *proximal* joint, which is farther from the front of the toe. When we talk about *mallet toes*, which are almost identical to hammer toes, we are referring to the *distal* joint, closer to the end of the toe. When both interphalangeal joints are contracted, the condition is called a *claw toe*. However, some health-care professionals use the terms interchangeably, and, rather than confuse the issue, I will confine my remarks primarily to the hammer toe, which is the most commonly used name for the contracture condition.

Actually, the mallet toe on the distal interphalangeal joint is dissimilar to the contracture on the proximal joint, in that it can be precipitated by tight shoes and/or tight hosiery to a far greater extent than a hammer toe, although the primary cause of both contractures is biomechanical. However, the symptoms, diagnosis, and treatment for both are basically identical.

DIAGRAM 5:3
Interphalangeal Joints

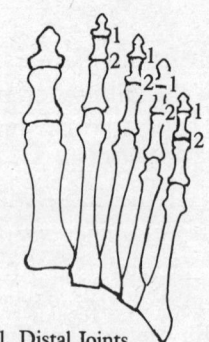

1. Distal Joints
2. Proximal Joints

Since the mallet-toe surgical procedure is virtually identical to hammer-toe surgical procedure, except that the mallet-toe procedure involves the distal interphalangeal joint, as opposed to the proximal interphalangeal joint in hammer toes, I shall only describe the hammer-toe procedure.

If we examine the biomechanics of the foot as they relate to the toes, we can understand how hammer toes develop. When the subtalar joint abnormally pronates, it creates excessive mobility in the forefoot—specifically in the *metatarso-phalangeal* joints (M.P.J.). As with bunions, one abnormally positioned bone forces another to also deviate. A *plantar-flexed metatarsal head* (a metatarsal bone whose head sits closer to the ground than that of any of the other metatarsals) will force the flexor digitorum longus and brevis tendons on the bottom of the toes to tighten as the corresponding muscles try to compensate for the abnormality and to keep the metatarsal bone and the toe bone (*phalanx*) aligned properly. When the muscles are pulled tight, the tendons at the ends of the muscles are also stretched to their limits. You will recall from our chapter on the anatomy of the foot that tendons are under stress whenever muscles are stretched beyond their limits. When the flexor digitorum longus (F.D.L.) muscles and their tendons are overstressed, the situation is similar to when a rope is attached at either end to something malleable. If the rope is pulled tight, the object begins to bend in or near the middle and bunch up. This is what happens with a toe that has overstressed muscles and tendons, and the end result is a hammer-shaped toe (remember Diagram 5:2).

Although a large number of the patients I see with hammer toes acquire the syndrome from a biomechanical fault, there are other causes as well. Most of the remainder do indeed result from constantly wearing shoes that do not fit properly. What usually happens is that a shoe that is too short, narrow, or shallow for the foot places constant abnormal pressure on the toes by causing them to contract or twist. Women who insist on wearing shoes with four-inch spike heels and constricting pointed toe-boxes are the most common examples of this. In fact, I have yet to meet a woman in this category who has gone five years without acquiring a deformed fifth toe.

The third most common cause of the hammer toe is a *pes cavus*, or *claw* foot. This is medicalese for an excessively arched foot that is almost S-curved (shown in Diagram 3:7). This excessive arch causes tightened tendons in the entire foot and usually results in the contracting of all five toes. A claw foot is usually congenital, but it can be caused on rare occasions by a neuro-muscular disease, or by a trauma that affects the neuro-muscular system of the foot. People who suffer from this condition have a difficult time finding shoes that are both comfortable and fashionable. I know this from experience, because my wife is such a person, and she is constantly complaining that she cannot find shoes she wants to wear.

The fourth, and rarest, cause of the hammer toe is neurological dysfunction in the foot, which can lead to contracture of the muscles and an abnormally high arch. Fortunately, I have seen few such cases in my years of podiatric practice. I say "fortunately" because these problems are generally quite difficult to treat. They are manifestations of systemic disorders that are often difficult to trace without expensive, uncomfortable, time-consuming testing. When these rare cases do occur, they are best referred to a neurologist for a complete neurological evaluation. Let me reassure you once again that neurological causes of hammer toes are indeed rare, and that they can be treated once the disorder is properly diagnosed.

In a lighter vein, I can definitely assure you that hammer toes are not caused by dropping heavy objects, such as hammers, on the front part of the foot, unless the pain from the injury causes you to walk abnormally for a very long period of time.

How the Hammer Toe Causes a Corn
Now that you know the causes of the hammer toe, we can once again turn our attention to the corn. Just keep in mind the shape of the toe once it has been affected by the tightening of the muscles and tendons: it is bent upwards at the first joint of the toe (Diagram 5:2).

Once the hammer toe is formed, wearing a normal shoe will begin to cause constant irritation to the elevated part of the toe. In order to prevent a serious inflammation from developing as a result of the irritation, a thickened layer of skin—a corn—will form on top of the toe.

If the corn were left alone, it would serve its protection purpose in peace and quiet. Unfortunately, however, the toe now has an even larger protuberance on the joint that is bent upwards. This situation makes wearing shoes even more of a problem, because the corn itself is being irritated, and that irritation touches the nerve endings under the skin. The pain eventually forces the person with the hammer toe to seek medical attention.

Actually, the problem is not always confined to the affected toe. In order to alleviate pain from a corn—without abandoning shoes that are ill-fitting—a person will compensate by altering his/her gait to avoid pressure on the offending toe. A person who walks abnormally can develop other biomechanical dysfunctions that could lead to problems in the lower limbs, and even in the lower back.

The Case of the Invisible Roots

The fact that corns can create indirect problems elsewhere in the body reminds me of one of my favorite cases—and of the many myths concerning the causes of cures and corns.

A few years ago a woman was referred to me by her family physician. She was suffering from knee pain that, according to her records, she believed to be caused by a corn on her second toe. When I asked how she arrived at that diagnosis, she replied immediately that the roots of her corn had wrapped themselves around the insides of her foot, all the way up her leg to her knee, thus providing the "root" cause of her knee pain.

I did my best to keep a straight face, and tried diplomatically to refute her theory. But she responded by insisting that I remove the corn, so that I could see for myself that its roots did indeed spread all the way up to her knee. To calm her, I did remove the corn tissue, and then tried to show her that no roots existed. However, she was far from convinced.

"The reason you can't see the roots," she said after some thought, "is that they are invisible. But I know you removed them as well. I can feel it."

The woman had no idea that my trimming of her corn was superficial, and, since she appeared to be relieved and satisfied, I did not attempt to reason with her further. She left my office quite pleased.

A few weeks later this same lady was back in my office, this time for the removal of an ingrown toenail. I curiously inquired as to the health of her knee, and was pleased to learn that within one week of the removal of her corn, her knee pain had disappeared.

This patient may have had the wrong diagnosis—corns definitely do not have roots—but she was quite accurate in assuming that her corn contributed greatly to her knee pain. As I mentioned above, when a corn, or any other foot disorder, causes pain in the foot, the sufferer, logically enough, begins to walk differently to remove pressure from the sore area. The altered gait produces either excessive pronation or excessive supination, either of which can result in knee pain. When the cause of the pain is removed, the reason for the abnormal gait is also eliminated, and the once-afflicted person returns to a normal biomechanical state when walking or running. Shortly thereafter, the knee pain will disappear. If it does not, the problem is probably not directly related to the foot.

Of course, my misinformed patient had no desire to learn the truth about her knee pain; she was adamant in sticking to her theory that the invisible corn-roots were the cause of her discomfort. I finally decided that if she was so convinced that corns have roots that can spread their tentacles up to the knee, why should I argue with her?

Treating Hammer Toes and Corns on Top of the Foot
As you know by now, a corn on top of the toe is caused by abnormal pressure on the toe joint that is bent upwards by the abnormal shape and positioning of the offending digit. That abnormal pressure is usually caused by a shoe that is too confined in the toe-box to allow space for the misshapen toe. So, how can we remove the corn, and thereby relieve the often excruciating pain that accompanies it? Well, as you might have guessed, there are conservative and invasive methods, and the treatment will often be determined by the general physical condition and age of the patient, the degree of dysfunction and discomfort, and the patient's life-style.

Home Remedies
Aside from my story about excising the mythical roots of a corn, there are a few other old wives' tales around about how to get rid of stubborn corns. Some of them even work, in rare cases, for reasons I will probably never understand. But I guarantee you that none of them will work permanently. Let me dwell on a few of them

briefly before getting to the more serious non-invasive forms of treatment.

A Vintage Cure

One of my favorite stories concerns a European patient of mine whom I had treated unsuccessfully for many months. I had tried all sorts of conservative measures, such as the constant trimming of the corn, the use of corn pads, the insertion of orthotics into his shoes, and his wearing of shoes with a larger toe-box. Just when I thought that surgery was the only way to remove the damned corn and its cause once and for all, he came into my office full of smiles. He just had to tell me that he had found an old French remedy that had worked wonders for him. Since I am a lover of fine wines, I found his story to be quite fascinating. Here it is: the red-wine cure for corns.

First the corn is soaked in warm water for twenty minutes. So far, so good. At the same time a corn pad is soaked in red wine, then in a ten-per-cent solution of salicylic acid. Then the corn pad is applied to the affected area, and left on for four days. After that time the foot is soaked again in warm water and, voilà, the corn is supposed to come out with ease. The same treatment can apparently be used for removing calluses, according to my patient, although the callus will not fall off after treatment. It will have to be gently pared down once it has been sufficiently softened by the concoction.

Of course, this concoction will not eliminate a biomechanical fault that caused the corn to develop, but it may indeed help alleviate discomfort caused by the corn, although my patient is the only person I know of who has tried it. Actually, I expect to see him hobbling into my office any day now, because I know the corn will eventually return. On the other hand, he may be content to keep on using this method of treatment, and, rather than correct the biomechanical fault in his foot, to live with the recurring corn. My only advice to people who might be interested in trying this method of treatment is to use the cheapest bottle of plonk you can find. Why waste expensive wine on your foot?

Beware of the Bottle

There are those people who make frequent purchases at their local pharmacies of small bottles of corn-remover. The problem with this supposedly magical cure is that it is made of a powerful acid that can burn away not only corns and calluses, but surrounding normal skin as well. Moreover, people often accept the principle that four drops are twice as effective as two. If this is the case, all they are doing is doubling their trouble. I treat about ten patients per month who have first-degree burns acquired from applying an extra-strength dose of corn-remover. Unfortunately, the majority of patients who fall into this category are older people, who seem to be more ready to accept home remedies, and less enthusiastic about seeking medical attention for their foot problems until they are in dire straits.

Too many of the elderly, and some of their juniors, also believe that if they cannot see the medication, it will not harm them. So they buy acid-treated pads to cover their corns, or the calluses on the bottom of their feet. In about ten days they remove the pad, along with the corn, plus healthy skin that has been burned off. They are left with a nastily infected skin ulcer that will require medical treatment.

The production and sale of corn pads and corn-removers has become a billion-dollar business over the years, and their use does provide temporary relief for minor cases of corns. But the corns will return as long as the underlying cause remains. And as the corn recurs, the person will increase the use of the acid treatments, often to the point where the skin has been burned right through to the underlying tissue. The fault lies not with the corn pad or the acid corn-remover, but with the user who is trying to eliminate the "root" problem. The burned skin and tissue will be exposed to bacterial infection as it ulcerates. That infection could result in severe medical complications, particularly in people suffering from systemic/circulatory conditions, such as diabetes.

Therefore, I strongly urge people who intend to use medicated corn pads and corn-remover liquids to apply them with discretion. If you are a diabetic or suffer from any kind of circulatory problem in your lower limbs, avoid them like the plague!

Don't Cut It Out!
Another home remedy that can have severe consequences is the use of a knife or a razor blade to perform "bathroom surgery" to cut

out a corn. Over the years, I have seen quite a few cases of people who took a shower or a bath, then used a sharp instrument to cut out a corn—along with a good deal of normal tissue. I can recall at least seven patients I had to stitch up after their clumsy attempts at bathroom surgery. A few of them actually reached the tendon before they discovered how deeply they had cut.

Conventional Conservative Approaches

A classic conservative approach to the treatment of corns, particularly those caused by hammer toes, would be to wear specially designed deep shoes that provide far more space for the forefoot than do regularly cut shoes. The extra room in the toe-box prevents the hammer toe from rubbing against the top of the shoe. It is that friction, you will recall, that causes the formation of the corn. The major problem with this approach is cosmetic. As an orthopedic surgeon colleague of mine once remarked, these so-called "orthopedic" shoes are made in only one model: black oxfords that people hate to wear because they are so ugly. Yet I strongly recommend them for people who have hammer toes but are poor candidates for surgical correction of their problem. I am referring mainly to those with poor circulation in their legs and feet, and those people who are elderly and generally not in the best of health. Orthopedic shoes are available in specialty stores throughout North America. Let me remind those of you who are reluctant to give up high-fashion footwear, despite discomfort, that it is far easier from a medical standpoint to change the shape of the shoe than it is to change the shape of the foot to fit an esthetically pleasing shoe.

Another conservative approach to alleviating the discomfort of a corn is the use of moisturizing creams and pumice stones, although they are generally beneficial only when "soft" corns are involved.

Moisturizing creams may, in fact, be better for the feet than for the face. An application morning and evening of any of the creams sold over cosmetic counters will work to keep corns soft and less painful.

The use of a pumice stone after showering or bathing will reduce the thickness of dead skin. This makes for more room for the toe inside the shoe and reduces pressure on the corn—and thus on the irritation. Just keep in mind that the creams and pumice stones will only alleviate the condition; the cause of the corn will still remain.

There is one conservative treatment that will be of some benefit to those people who are poor surgical risks and who ought to avoid medicated corn pads and corn-removal liquids at all costs. It involves the use of a *buttress pad*. This pad elevates the offending toe, as it slips both over and under it. The pad cushions the toe from above and below, and also serves to straighten out mild hammer-toe conditions. The application of this buttress pad, along with monthly trimming of the corn by an expert, will alleviate much of the discomfort, and ought to be the prime form of treatment for those people who are generally most at risk from surgical intervention and the use of acid-based pads. Those who most often fall into this category are the elderly.

Surgical Remedies for the Hammer Toe and the Corn

For some people the surgical approach is the best answer. In this category are people who are unable or unwilling to put up with a certain amount of discomfort, and who demand immediate relief without having to change the style of shoes they wear.

There are many new techniques for treating the hammer toe, and the corn that develops on top of the toe because of it. The least involved is called the *soft-tissue release*, or the *plantar set*, procedure. There is a minimal amount of trauma to the area caused by the incision, although people with diabetic and/or circulatory problems may still be poor candidates for the operation. This technique can be used successfully only when the two tendons above and below the bone are tight in the area of the hammer toe but the bones themselves are normal. This is most often the case in the early stages of the development of a hammer toe.

The soft-tissue release is a minimal-incision (M.I.S.) procedure done under a local anesthetic, usually in a doctor's office. A tiny instrument is used to cut the offending tendon(s) via the underside of the deformed toe. Once the tendons have been cut, the toe automatically straightens out, eliminating the hammer shape. Although they have been severed, these cut tendons will eventually lengthen and reattach to themselves without further medical intervention. It takes from six to twelve months for that to happen. Usually the incision is so small that stitches are not required, and post-operative discomfort is minimal. The success rate for this procedure is quite high.

The soft-tissue-release operation normally works quite well as long as no bone in the area has been deformed. If there is a bone deformity, the technique is ill-advised, since the toe will still not straighten out. If a bone is involved, the surgeon must proceed to Plan B.

Plan B involves a procedure called *arthroplasty*, a word that means "surgically remodelling a joint". Arthroplasty can be done either "closed" or "open", depending on the condition of the toe joint and/or the technique preferred by the surgeon.

The Operation Was a Success, But the Patient Wouldn't Follow the Rules of the Recovery Game

While it is vital for the surgeon to bandage and position the toe properly after the operation, it is equally important for the patient to ensure that the proper bandaging, or splinting, of the toe is maintained until the healing process has been completed. Usually the healing process will take a couple of weeks; however, this depends on the severity of the deformity that was corrected, and the patient's general physical condition. In a complicated operation, the recovery time will be longer, and splinting of the toe may be required for up to two months. It is essential, therefore, for the doctor to explain precisely, and clearly, to the patient what must be done and what must be avoided to ensure a successful outcome of the treatment. Once again, "communication" becomes a key word.

Communication between doctor and patient is also important before surgery so that the patient understands that when the operation has been successfully completed, the toe from which the offending corn was removed will be slightly shorter if part of the proximal phalanx had to be removed. Or, in the case of a soft-tissue-release procedure, the newly shaped toe will appear to be slightly longer because the offending tendon(s) will have been cut, thereby releasing the pulling effect on the toe joint. Many patients, unaware of the new shape of their surgically treated toe, have become needlessly frightened because they thought the operation was intended to make the toe perfectly symmetrical with the others. Such is not the case. What the surgeon has done is to remove the cause of the irritation and return the foot to a condition where weight-bearing is properly distributed on the foot. As a result, it should not be necessary after such surgery to require the wearing of an orthotic device, even though the foot continues to over-pronate. The biomechanical fault no longer adversely affects the toe.

It will be necessary, however, after hammer-toe and corn-removal surgery, for the patient to wear proper shoes so that the toes are not scrunched together and/or irritated again by shoes that are too shallow for the foot. Remember that in a few cases, ill-fitting shoes can themselves be the cause of a hammer toe and a corn.

Soft-Core Corn

So far in this chapter I have concentrated primarily on the causes and treatment of corns that sit on top of the toes. These are hard layers of dead, thickened skin that form to protect the irritated part of a hammer toe from becoming even more inflamed. However, corns also form on the sides of the toes, and, because they are somewhat moistened by perspiration between the toes, they are called "soft" or "wet" corns (*heloma molle*, in medicalese). But, despite their name, they are hard—much harder than normal skin—and they can be far more painful than corns on top of the toes because of their proximity to nerves that run along the inside of the toes. The friction caused by toe rubbing against corn can irritate these nerves fiercely. And if one is unlucky enough to have corns on adjacent sides of two toes, and those corns are constantly rubbing against each other, the discomfort can be multiplied exponentially. By the way, these adjacent corns have been dubbed "kissing corns" by a colleague of mine, who hastens to add that they are not caused by having a sexual partner with a foot fetish.

Whatever these soft corns are called, there is no mistaking the fact that they are a pain in the foot. They are usually caused by a bony growth, which causes the toe to jut out, and this results in friction with the adjacent toe (see Diagram 5:4). The condition is exacerbated by wearing shoes that are too tight in the front. Once the soft corn has fully flowered, even properly fitting shoes will cause irritation, because the inflamed area is so exquisitely sore that even a minor amount of friction will result in the nerves in the toe being irritated.

DIAGRAM 5:4
The Formation of a Soft Corn

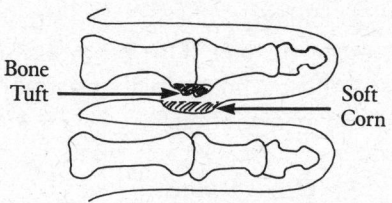

Although it is obvious that scrunched toes are squeezed together by tight shoes, it is not quite so clear why the bony deformity that causes the corn to develop occurs in the first place. It is generally thought to be caused by a biomechanical fault combined with too tight a shoe, which forces the offending toe to curl sideways. Instead of being transformed into a hammer toe, the offending toe is forced to lie up against an adjacent toe in an awkward position. As in the development of a bunion, the bone is forced to jut out. It then becomes irritated, and subsequently a corn forms to protect it.

Soft-Corn Treatment
If the soft corn is newly developed and quite mild, the treatment is quite simple. The corn is trimmed and a donut pad is applied to protect the area. At the same time the patient is strongly urged to switch to more comfortable shoes to avoid further problems. Unfortunately, not all my patients comply with the suggestion that they wear better-fitting shoes.

For my recalcitrant patients, I am eventually obliged to take more vigorous action to treat their soft corns. I also see patients for the first time who have soft-corn problems that are beyond the stage of non-surgical treatment. Rest assured, though, that surgery for these types of corns is minor, and is done using an M.I.S. technique that does not involve much time or discomfort on the part of the patient.

The procedure is called *exostectomy*, and it involves shaving down the protruding bone with a burr that has been introduced through a small stab incision in the toe. The surgery is done in a doctor's office under a local anesthetic, and requires only a stitch or two to close the wound made by the incision. The patient can then walk fairly easily out of the office after the operation and return to his/ her normal activity, as long as it does not require a lot of time spent on the feet for the rest of the day. This procedure is done by almost all foot surgeons, even those who normally use only open techniques, because it is quite a simple operation.

Between a Nail and a Hard Place

One other type of corn that can be a real pain is the *subungal heloma* (medicalese for "corn under the nail"). It is caused by a small tuft of bone that forms at the end of the toe bone under the nail (see Diagram 5:5). This bone tuft develops either because of a trauma to the offending bone—particularly in the case of youngsters—or as a result of some hereditary quirk.

DIAGRAM 5:5
The Formation of a Corn Under a Toenail

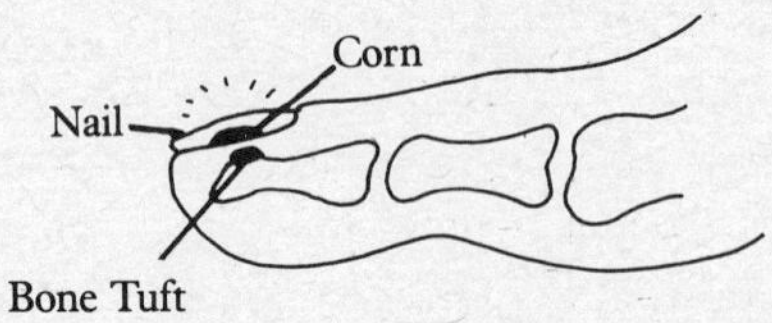

I will see at least one patient per month with this problem, and the common complaint is of pain in the nail area of the affected toe. The patient will say that it feels like an ingrown nail, or as if something is growing under the nail. The reason for this is the direct pressure being brought to bear on the soft tissue between the tuft of bone and the nail. This pressure is being caused by the tissue being squeezed in a cramped space, often by shoes that may be too tight. To help alleviate this sensitivity, and to protect the bone tuft, a corn forms under the nail bed, where the pressure is being felt. Because of the growth of the corn, the space between the bone tuft and the nail becomes even more cramped. As a result the pain increases.

The condition can occasionally be relieved by a simple change of footwear. It is possible to avoid irritating the area if a person wears shoes that fit properly in the toe-box. However, most of the time the problem has been allowed to develop over a long period of time, either because it was mis-diagnosed as a fungal nail, or something similar, or because the diagnosis was hypochondria—an all too common occurrence.

There are two ways of treating the subungal heloma, if a simple change of footwear fails to provide relief. If the condition appears to have been caused by an isolated, traumatic incident, the solution is to remove the corn surgically. This can be done in a doctor's office under a local anesthetic, and the patient will be ambulatory immediately after the corn has been removed. The operation involves removing an overlying piece of nail, then excising the corn beneath it.

If the corn recurs repeatedly, the bone tuft itself should be removed. This can also be done in a doctor's office under a local anesthetic. Discomfort to the patient is minimal, and he or she ought to be able to walk easily out of the office after the operation has been completed. This procedure involves a small incision through a side, or the end, of the offending toe. A surgical instrument, usually a burr, is then introduced through this incision, and the tuft of bone is filed down. The nail itself is left untouched. The success rate with this type of closed procedure is almost one hundred per cent. Foot surgeons are in general agreement in this case that the M.I.S. technique is the procedure of choice.

Baby Blues
The baby, or fifth, toe is particularly susceptible to corns, both hard and soft. Most of the time the corns, which may develop on the top or on either side of the toe, are created by shoe pressure: there is simply too little space in the toe-box to accommodate the baby toe, which is then twisted and contracts over a period of years until it appears that the top of the toe is actually on the outside (see Diagram 5:6). This condition is called an *axially rotated toe*.

An axially rotated baby toe is biomechanically unsound, and it is also being squeezed by a tight shoe on its outside, and by the toe next to it. As a result, corns develop, and they can be excruciatingly painful—as many of my patients are all too eager to tell me. Baby-

DIAGRAM 5:6
An Axially Rotated Fifth Toe

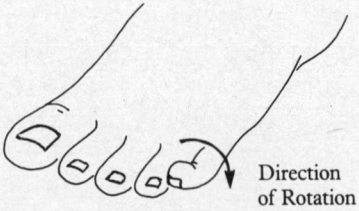

Direction
of Rotation

toe corns appear most commonly on the top or outside of the toe, and less frequently on the inside of the toe. In any case, the treatment is similar.

If the wearing of more comfortably fitting shoes and/or corn pads does not sufficiently alleviate the discomfort, surgery will be required. Once again it can easily be done in a doctor's office under a local anesthetic. Basically, the axially rotated baby toe will have to be *de-rotated*, that is, turned back into its normal shape.

In this procedure, a semi-lunar incision is made, and the head of the proximal phalanx (the largest bone in the toe) of the baby toe is excised. The toe is then rotated back to its normal position, using a skin-flapping technique. The patient will suffer little discomfort following the operation, and will be immediately ambulatory. Assuming that the surgery was properly done, and that the patient followed the post-operation-care rules, recovery will take no more than a few days.

6

Coming to the Fore: Problems of the Front of the Foot

Forefoot Facts

As you will remember from Chapter Two, the forefoot is composed of: the five metatarsal bones; the two phalanges (bones) in the great toe, and the three phalanges in the other toes; the *sesamoid* bones behind the metatarsals; the joints; the soft tissue such as muscles, tendons, ligaments, and other connective tissue; the nerves; and the veins, arteries, and smaller blood vessels that provide the area with a steady fresh supply of nutrients.

The forefoot is the workhorse of the foot, because it is in contact with the ground seventy-five per cent of the time during the stance phase of the gait cycle (that is, when you are in stride). Therefore, it receives the majority of the pounding to which the foot is subjected when a person is walking, running, or doing other stressful things while upright.

Unlike the rearfoot and the midfoot, which have a few very solid bone structures, the forefoot has twenty-one bones that work together intricately to help propel the leg forward. So it is not surprising that more can go wrong with the forefoot than with the rest of the foot, particularly when weight distribution on the bottom of the foot is normally far greater at the front.

Yet, considering the odds against the forefoot, it is surprising that less than five per cent of the North American population will ever break a toe, and less than one per cent will ever fracture a metatarsal bone. This is an amazing fact, considering what klutzes some

75

of us are, and the lengths to which many of us go to wear improper footwear, but it has been recently documented. The most common problems involving the forefoot are calluses and corns, and we have dealt with these conditions in other chapters. However, there are other disorders affecting the forefoot that can be quite interesting, and distressing, and we will discuss them in this chapter. Most of them involve inflammations of tendons, ligaments, joints, and nerves, but a few of them concern fractures of the many bones in the forefoot.

I have already described a typical conversation between a doctor and a patient involving foot pain. The doctor told the patient that the problem was *metatarsalgia*. The patient became anxious because the word sounded ominous. But you know now that all "metatarsalgia" means is a "pain in the area of the metatarsal bones in the forefoot". In essence the doctor is merely agreeing with the patient that he/she has a sore forefoot, and nothing else.

Now, if you went to a doctor and told him that you had a tummy-ache, and were informed after a cursory examination that you had a "sore stomach", would you be satisfied with the diagnosis? I should hope not, particularly if the doctor tells you that it will clear up quickly by itself, or that an operation ought to be performed to investigate. Well, the same applies to the forefoot. Never settle for a diagnosis of "metatarsalgia", because it means nothing. If a doctor tells you that your foot pain will magically disappear on its own, or that the foot ought to be dissected to better evaluate the situation, run as fast as you can out of the office in search of another opinion.

There are distinct reasons for metatarsalgia that involve inflammation and/or fractures of a bone, as well as a whole host of soft-tissue problems, and the treatments must obviously vary with the disorder. One thing to keep in mind here, as compared to the analogy of the tummy-ache, is that forefoot pain is almost never indicative of any major disease, and that the cause of the pain is rarely terribly difficult to treat.

A Metatarsal-Head Ache

One of the problems a foot doctor faces when he has a patient who complains of pain in the area of the metatarsals is properly diagnosing the condition. There are many disorders that have symptoms that mimic each other, and it takes an expert to determine the actual cause of the discomfort. Let us examine one of the most common conditions: *metatarsal-head pain*, which is the third-most-common cause of visits to my office, after calluses and corns, and ingrown toenails.

The Causes of a Metatarsal-Head Ache

One of the causes of a metatarsal-head pain is the *plantar-flexed* metatarsal bone (see Diagram 3:8). The plantar-flexed metatarsal does not drop down as we walk, it is always down. It sits lower than the other metatarsal heads which naturally rise and drop during the normal gait cycle. As a result, the plantar-flexed metatarsal bone is always bearing shock by itself, directly on the end of its head. Why the metatarsal bone becomes plantar-flexed is still medical conjecture, but the problem is exacerbated by ill-fitting shoes, particularly those that have very thin soles with little cushion for absorbing shock during walking or running. That shock often winds up being absorbed by the metatarsal heads. By the time metatarsal-head pain has begun, even comfortable, shock-absorbing shoes will probably be of little help. The reason is that once the metatarsal head has become swollen and inflamed, only total elimination of the irritation will calm down the area.

The heads of the metatarsal bones form joints with the *proximal phalanges* (the largest bones in the toes). A plantar-flexion will cause irritation at the offending joint. This irritation can take the form of either *capsulitis* or *synovitis*. A *capsule* is a lining on the outside of a joint; a *synovium* is a lining on the inside of a joint. Hence we have the terms capsulitis and synovitis to describe inflammations of these linings. In this case, the inflammation is of the linings of the metatarso-phalangeal joint.

The major symptom of these types of inflammation is the sensation of a bad bruise to a bone in the area of the trouble, almost as if the sufferer had stepped on a stone. Unfortunately, this symptom is somewhat similar to that experienced by someone suffering from a *neuroma* (a nerve condition discussed later in this chapter), because the inflamed area is very close to the interspace through which the nerve passes.

Our old friend, abnormal pronation, is also a prime cause of metatarsal-head pain. Unlike plantar-flexion, however, it does not involve just one faulty metatarsal bone; the biomechanical fault is spread widely across the entire foot.

As you know, when a foot pronates, the weight on the foot cuts across the metatarsal heads from the baby toe over to the big toe. Each metatarsal head is subjected to weight at slightly different times, rather than together with the others. Therefore, while a person is walking or running, each head is absorbing one hundred per cent of the weight of the body for a brief interval. That places tremendous stress on each metatarsal head with every step.

You may also recall that when a foot pronates, it "rolls" from the outside in. Something has to stop that roll; otherwise you would look very strange if you over-pronated badly, for you would be constantly turning or twisting your foot as you completed your step. What happens is that the big toe provides the support to break the "roll". The foot widens and forces the big toe to angle inwards. The result is the tandem of the first and second metatarsal heads acting together to absorb enough of the force to halt the roll. If a person over-pronates significantly, the second metatarsal head receives a large amount of the abnormal force and becomes inflamed; the big toe angles further inwards and eventually the detour causes a bunion.

This action can produce metatarsal-head pain in the second metatarsal bone, and the discomfort is quite similar symptomatically to plantar-flexion-induced pain, and therefore is also difficult to distinguish from neuroma-induced pain. To complicate matters even further, it is possible, though uncommon, to suffer from both a neuroma and metatarsal-head pain at the same time. The proximity of the metatarsal heads to the nerves passing through the interspaces can result in one inflammation triggering another. For example, a metatarsal head that is inflamed will cause swelling around the nerve. That swelling may eventually constrict the space through which the nerve must pass, thereby setting up the possible development of a neuroma. At that point, the symptoms will mimic those of both a neural and a metatarsal-head problem. This will complicate both diagnosis and treatment of the conditions, as you can imagine.

There has been much speculation as to what comes first, the metatarsal-head disorder or the neuroma. In my opinion, it is usually the metatarsal-head inflammation that will result in the development of the nerve inflammation, although the reverse is definitely possible.

I have had excellent success over the years diagnosing these disorders, and determining which of the conditions exist. I will be describing below how I test for nerve inflammation. My basic technique for establishing the existence of metatarsal-head pain is by *palpating* (using my hands and fingertips to probe the affected area) *directly over* the metatarsal head. If this palpating produces pain, I can be reasonably secure in my diagnosis, particularly if the tests for a neuroma are negative.

Heading Off the Villain

How do we treat metatarsal-head pain that has been caused by a biomechanical fault in the foot? You guessed it—by using an orthotic device to correct the fault, and with the injection or oral use of an anti-inflammatory drug to alleviate the inflammation if it is severe. Although the problem is often one of abnormal shock-absorption stress on the metatarsal heads, the use of simple shock-absorption pads does not correct the metatarsal-head weight-distribution problem. If the condition is not too severe, I will use a simple *padding-and-taping* technique to reposition the weight on the affected metatarsal head (see Diagram 6:1). This procedure works best with a mild plantar-flexed metatarsal bone that is inflamed because of an injury to the area.

DIAGRAM 6:1
Padding and Taping

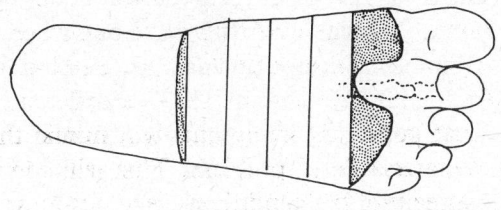

Quarter-Inch Felt Pad Held
On by Tape

When the condition is chronic, either with a plantar-flexed toe or abnormal pronation, I will suggest the use of an orthotic device that will resolve the weight-distribution problem on the metatarsal heads. The orthotic will have to be worn at all times, since neither condition will cure itself once a person is fully grown.

If a temporary problem has arisen out of a traumatic injury, such as stepping on a stone or a similar object, the padding-and-taping technique will probably work quite well. At the same time, ultra-sound and/or a cortisone injection may help to relieve the temporary inflammation. As much as I hate to use anti-inflammatory drugs—either cortisone injections or non-steroidal pills—there are situations where a cortisone shot will definitely help relieve the inflammation in the forefoot.

Surgery is also a last resort for treatment of metatarsal-head pain. However, if the metatarsal head is severely dropped down, and is causing all sorts of mischief, such as painful calluses under the head, a *metatarsal osteotomy* may be the only way to permanently correct the problem. This procedure involves breaking the metatarsal bone and repositioning it to allow for a normal metatarsal-head function. It is not as gruesome as it sounds, and can produce excellent results with a minimum of discomfort during the healing stage, providing the patient follows post-operative-care instructions.

Of course, there are problems with an osteotomy regardless of whether it involves metatarsal bones or any other bones in the body. The major concern is that of *non-union* of the bones broken by a surgical procedure. The desired effect of an osteotomy is to have a problem corrected by the surgical breaking of a bone so that the part of the body involved can be realigned properly. In normal circumstances, the severed ends of the bone will rejoin naturally over a period of time and you will eventually have one whole bone again, but one that is biomechanically normal, without undue stress on the metatarsal head. However, occasionally the floating end of the metatarsal bone will not reunite with the rest of the bone. This "divorce" is called a *non-union*. It is more prevalent in older people, who tend to "baby" their feet more after surgery by not walking enough. Unexercised bones will lose calcium and refuse to heal properly after a period of time. When this happens, the two pieces of bone will have to be fused, either with the introduction of bone chips—usually taken from the hip—to the area to rejoin bone to bone, or with the aid of a newer technique, *electromagnetic therapy*, that is still in experimental stages.

The second problem with an osteotomy of a metatarsal bone is that the floating end of the bone may move abnormally high and cause a problem with an adjacent metatarsal bone (see Diagram 6:2) If, for example, the floating piece of the second metatarsal bone sits so high that there is no longer any weight on its head, the third metatarsal head will then be subjected to the brunt of body weight distributed in that area when a person is in stride. This happens about twenty per cent of the time after an osteotomy of a metatarsal bone. Naturally, the third metatarsal head becomes inflamed because of the added weight it must bear, until it eventually requires medical treatment—perhaps an osteotomy of its own. Actually, a foot surgeon could make a living off the same foot by chasing metatarsal-head pain from one end of the foot to the other, and then back again to the beginning. However, this would be most unusual.

DIAGRAM 6:2
Cross-Section of Metatarsal Heads, Showing Weight Shift from Second to Third Head

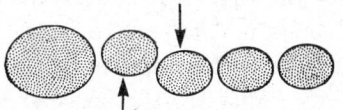

A Bad Case of Nerves
We have already spoken of nerve disorders in the forefoot. Let us now discuss them in greater detail, particularly *neuromas*.

A neuroma is a benign tumor of a nerve caused by an abnormal growth of nerve cells in response to an irritation. Let me emphasize that a neuroma in the forefoot is never more than a simple irritated pinched nerve that has erupted because of constant compression and irritation—either between metatarsal heads, or at the base of the proximal phalanges (the largest bones in the toes). You can see the area where neuromas are most likely to occur in Diagram 6:3.

DIAGRAM 6:3
Articulation of Metatarsal Bones and Some Resultant Problems

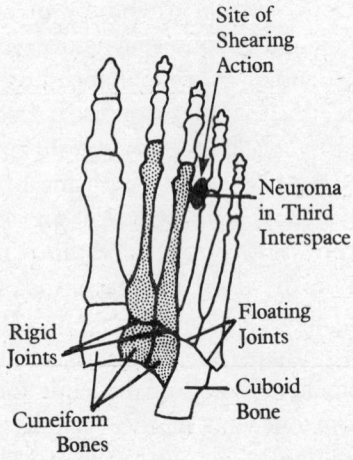

A neuroma may develop when poor biomechanical function of a foot causes a chronic irritation of a nerve, thereby triggering the growth of additional nerve cells. The extra nerve tissue is nature's way of trying to protect the nerve from further irritation; but the opposite occurs because a vicious cycle develops. The extra nerve tissue takes up space and forces further irritation, because it is now even closer to the offending bone structure. Then, as the nerve becomes further inflamed, it develops more tissue to protect its core and therefore further compresses the space through which it must pass. This merry-go-round continues until the sufferer is required to seek medical attention, because the discomfort has become too extreme to ignore.

As I mentioned above, faulty biomechanics of the foot are the major cause of a neuroma. The second most likely cause, which often acts in conjunction with the first, is the wearing of ill-fitting shoes that squeeze the forefoot and also force it to accept almost all of the body's weight during walking or running. The worst culprits are ladies' high-heeled shoes. The third possible cause of a neuroma is a swelling of the foot, for whatever reason, that serves to reduce the space through which the nerves must pass. The fourth, and least common, cause is an abnormal bony structure or growth that also pinches the nerve as it tries to pass through the areas normally reserved for its passage.

Aside from the causes I have mentioned, there are two theories that attempt to explain more clinically the cause of the neuroma. I will try to explain them as best I can without resorting to excessive medicalese.

The first theory is that there is a difference in the way the second and third metatarsal bones *articulate* (meet to form a joint) with the cuneiform bones behind them, and the way the fourth and fifth metatarsal bones articulate with the cuboid bone behind them (see Diagram 6:3). The second and third metatarsal bones form a basically rigid joint with their respective cuneiform bones; the fourth and fifth metatarsal bones form a movable joint with the cuboid bone. In a sense, the fourth and fifth metatarsals float, and the action of the fourth, compared to that of the rigid third metatarsal, results in a sharing effect at the third interspace between the third and fourth metatarsals. Therefore, when the fourth metatarsal bone shears down (also shown in Diagram 6:3), it cuts at the space through which the nerve passes. Naturally, the nerve may then become irritated, and a neuroma may develop.

To understand the second theory, you have to recall the path of the *tibialis posterior nerve* that splits into the *medial* and *lateral plantar nerves* once it enters the foot itself. The medial nerve runs along the bottom of the foot to the big-toe side, while the lateral nerve travels along the bottom of the foot to the baby-toe side.

As it approaches the area of the metatarsal bones, the medial plantar nerve branches out, one twig passing through the first interspace between the toes, the next one through the second interspace, and the third through the third interspace. The lateral plantar nerve branches into two twigs—one passing through the fourth interspace, the other through the third. If you have been counting, you will have quickly realized that two separate, tiny nerves run through the third interspace (see Diagram 6:4). So there is a double thickness of nerve there, hence the greater frequency of neuromas occurring at the third interspace. Whoever designed the foot apparently did not compensate adequately enough for this extra amount of nerve tissue in the area.

DIAGRAM 6:4
Plantar Nerves

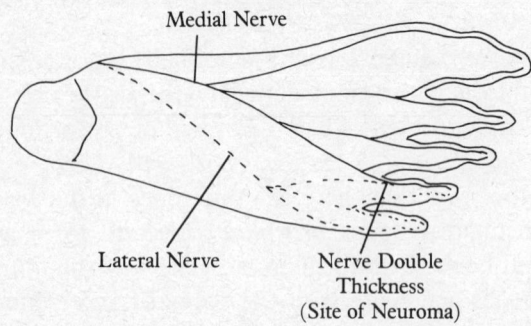

Medial Nerve

Lateral Nerve   Nerve Double
Thickness
(Site of Neuroma)

Lending credence to this second theory is the fact that the most common site of a forefoot neuroma is at the *third* interspace, between the third and fourth toes. In descending order are neuromas of the second interspace, the first, and, lastly, the fourth. The most common one was first identified by Dr. Dudley Morton, an early pioneer in foot-disorders research, and the man responsible for the dubious existence of the *Morton's toe syndrome*. As a consequence, a neuroma in the third interspace has for years been called *Morton's neuroma*.

The symptoms of a forefoot neuroma will generally vary from patient to patient, and can range from mild to severe. The most common symptom is a burning sensation in the area of the neuroma. This may be accompanied by a feeling of pins and needles in the affected toes. Some patients will actually experience a popping or dislocating sensation in the interspace involved. Many people with the disorder will also feel a generalized ache and pain in the offending interspace, sometimes accompanied by the unpleasant feeling of a hot knife cutting through the bottom of the foot. The discomfort will inevitably be exacerbated by the wearing of shoes that are too tight, particularly those with high heels that force extra weight onto the forefoot.

One of the tests that I use to determine the presence of a neuroma is called *Mulder's sign*, after the doctor who invented the diagnostic procedure. The right thumb of the clinician is placed under the involved interspace and the left hand is used to squeeze together the metatarsal heads. If a neuroma is there, it will create a popping sensation, and the patient will probably curse loudly, questioning your ancestry in the process, since the painful symptoms of the disorder will be reproduced by the squeezing. The bigger the pop, the larger the neuroma. The test is about eighty-five per cent effective in distinguishing neuromas from metatarsal-head pain.

Treating the Nervous Breakdown of the Foot
Unfortunately, I cannot give you a one-hundred-per-cent guarantee when it comes to the treatment of a neuroma. The best I can do is cite a seventy-five-per-cent success rate when it comes to treating the problem, regardless of the cause or the treatment method.

The treatment is based on the cause of the disorder. If the problem has been caused by improper footwear, the obvious thing to do first is to change shoes permanently. At the same time, if the neuroma is causing the patient a lot of discomfort, I may opt for an injection of cortisone with an anesthetic into the area around the inflamed nerve. Relief may occur in about thirty per cent of the cases, although initially, for a couple of days, the discomfort may actually increase, because the injection itself can irritate the nerve. If the cortisone injection fails to relieve the discomfort, I may then try a shot of cortisone plus vitamin B_{12}. Vitamin B_{12} is an anti-*neuritis* (inflammation of a nerve) medication. Unfortunately, the success rate with the combination of medications is also only thirty per cent.

If the cause of the neuroma is determined to be biomechanical, a *metatarsal support* can be used (see Diagram 6:5). It serves to widen the space between the third and fourth metatarsal bones, thereby increasing the area of the third interspace that the nerves must pass through. Should the biomechanical fault be one of abnormal pronation, an orthotic device can be prescribed. The orthotic will correct the abnormal pronation and also provide for the proper weight distribution at the metatarsal heads.

DIAGRAM 6:5
Metatarsal Support

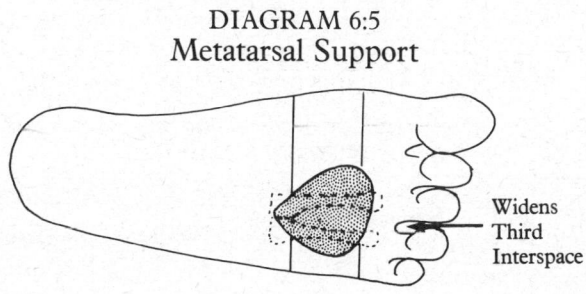

Widens
Third
Interspace

If the neuroma is severe enough to drastically restrict the regular activities of the patient, I may consider surgery. However, I would choose this path only if the patient's quality of life was abysmal because of the discomfort. I am most reluctant to perform nerve surgery, because it is tricky and does not always provide the desired effect.

I can recall the time when a female patient of mine was accompanied by her husband to my office for an examination of her severe Morton's neuroma. I told her that because her life-style was restricted by the excruciating pain caused by the neuroma, surgery was an option for her.

"I'll try anything," she exclaimed, before I even had a chance to explain what was involved with the surgery and what the complications might be. "I can't even go shopping any more, my foot hurts so much when I walk."

At that point her husband rolled his eyes and then glanced sideways at me, trying to whisper that I should not encourage the operation. I quickly asked the woman to put on her shoes and stockings while I waited outside the examining room with her husband.

"Why don't you want her to have the operation?" I asked him softly.

"Because," he whispered, "if she starts running loose again in the stores, we'll be broke by the end of the year."

Fortunately the woman eventually did respond to a cortisone injection and orthotics, sparing me a moral dilemma.

Surgery for a severely inflamed neuroma involves the removal of the affected portion of the nerve. It can be done in a doctor's office under a local anesthetic, and it takes about a half-hour to perform. The patient is immediately ambulatory, and ought to be completely recovered after ten to fourteen days. During the recovery period, the discomfort should be only a tiny fraction of what it was before the neuroma was removed. In fact, one patient of mine was out playing golf three days after the surgery, and hardly noticed any discomfort at all. She told me that by the end of the game she had totally forgotten about the operation and the neuroma she once had. However, her amazing recovery is most unusual.

March Break: The Stress Fracture
It used to be common in the United States Marine Corps to test

the mettle of new recruits by sending them out on twenty-mile runs after only a short period of boot-camp training. The recruits would be forced to wear army boots rather than running shoes, in order to make the test a bit more sadistic. You try running twenty miles when out of shape, and when forced to wear heavy boots. In about five per cent of the recruits a phenomenon was observed: so-called *march fractures* of a metatarsal bone, caused by the stress of the run in abnormal running footwear. We are more familiar with the condition by its more common name, *stress fracture*. The metatarsal bone most likely to be involved is the second (fifty per cent of the time); next is the third (twenty-five per cent of the time); the other twenty-five per cent of the cases involve the fourth metatarsal. I have never seen a stress fracture of either the first or the fifth metatarsal bones.

A stress fracture of a bone is caused by excessive, often continuous, pressure on a part of the bone during a given time, particularly over a lengthy period. It is fairly common, medically speaking, in metatarsal bones, but can occur in most of the bones in the foot and lower leg. Novice Marines are not the only people susceptible to the condition. It also affects a lot of runners who overstress one part of their feet for various reasons, aerobic exercisers who partake to excess, and women who walk long distances in high-heeled shoes that place extra pressure on the forefoot. A metatarsal bone can also be stress-fractured as a foot attempts to deal naturally with a plantar-flexion problem. Once the plantar-flexed metatarsal has broken on its own, it will be quite sore, but weight distribution on the metatarsal heads should become fairly normal.

One would imagine that a fracture would show up clearly enough on an X-ray, but such is not the case with a stress fracture—unless it is quite severe—until about four to six weeks have elapsed from the time of the break. When it does show up on an X-ray, what is seen is the bone-healing *callus* (*bone callus*), which forms around fractured bone-ends and is essential in the healthy reuniting of the ends of the bone.

So, if a stress fracture does not show up on an X-ray, how is it diagnosed? One way is to palpate the shaft of the metatarsal bone. If pain is produced by pressing on the offending part of the bone, you become suspicious. Also, the area on the top of the metatarsal bone will be quite swollen if a break has occurred. In some instances, where diagnosis is difficult, a *bone scan* is done. If the radioactive dye, which is painlessly injected into the bloodstream, shows a "hot spot" where a break is suspected, it is generally a confirmation of the diagnosis. We see about six metatarsal stress fractures per week at our Sports Medicine Clinic, but we are reluctant to order bone scans unless we find diagnosis difficult, or if the suspected break has not shown signs of healing eight to nine weeks after the injury, despite the proper treatment. As you might have guessed, it may be difficult at times to distinguish a metatarsal stress-fracture from other forefoot problems if the symptons are not clear-cut.

Stress-Fracture Treatment

A fracture, be it of the stress variety or of the type caused by a severe traumatic incident, will normally heal on its own. Unlike fractures of other bones in the body, the metatarsals, however, do not require immobilization in a plaster cast, because they are not put out of alignment by the stress fracture. Therefore, a cast is not required to hold the mending bone in the proper position. This fact makes it easier to live with during the recovery period.

However, the damaged bone must not be stressed further by carrying on with any activities that put excess pressure on the forefoot—that is, with the type of activity that caused the fracture in the first place. Those types of activities would include running, playing racquet sports, and undertaking similar athletic endeavors. Also, do not wear high-heeled shoes that also put extra stress on the forefoot. Comfortable running-shoes are the perfect footwear for the normal eight-to-twelve-week recovery period.

Ultrasound treatment is definitely *not* recommended for a stress fracture. Ultrasound seems to interfere with the natural healing process of broken bones. I have seen a few patients who have related to me the suffering they underwent from pain produced by ultra-sound treatment that was wrongfully prescribed. The problem is not with uneducated therapists, it is with the initial mis-diagnosis of the problem. Stress fractures, as I mentioned above, can be easily mistaken for other metatarsal disorders.

Finally, use a bit of common sense. If you have been diagnosed as having a metatarsal stress-fracture, you will have to exercise a bit of patience until the break has healed on its own. If you try to push yourself—for example, by running too soon or wearing high heels before the break has healed—you will compound your suffering and push back the date of your recovery by a few weeks.

The Sesamoid Bones

As you can see from Diagram 6:6, there are two bones, the *sesamoids*, that sit under the first metatarsal bone at the big-toe joint. Since there seems to be little use for these sesame-seed-shaped bones vis-à-vis the biomechanics of the foot, they are thought to be remnants, according to evolutionary theory, of our ancestors, who may have spent more time on all fours than most of us do nowadays.

DIAGRAM 6:6
Sesamoid Bones and the Nerve Involved in Sesamoiditis

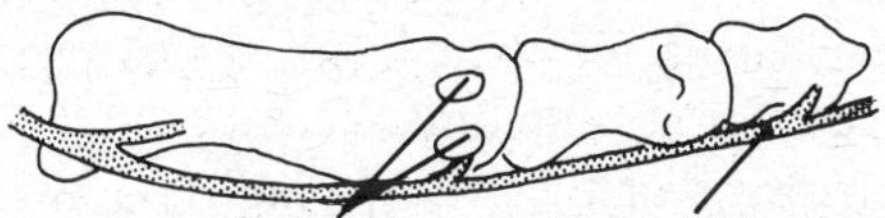

Underside of the Big
Toe

Sesamoids   Proper Digital Nerve

Although the sesamoid bones play a *tiny* role in the biomechanics of the human foot, the same is not true for horses. Sesamoid fractures are not uncommon in race horses, because of the pounding the equine hoof takes while the horse is running, and when that unfortunate break occurs, the horse sometimes has to be destroyed. However, that is not to say that humans are able to avoid sesamoid problems—the solution is just considerably less drastic.

Sesamoid bones can fracture, unfortunately, and the soft tissue around the bones can become painfully inflamed. The reason for this is twofold. First, the sesamoid bones sit very close to the surface of the foot. Secondly, they are often exposed directly to the ground by a plantar-flexed first metatarsal bone. This condition is called a *forefoot valgus deformity* (remember Diagram 3:4). While the deformity itself does not cause discomfort or dysfunction, it does expose the sesamoid bones to undue stress that can lead to problems in the area.

Sesamoiditis

Sesamoiditis is an inflammation of the area under the first metatarsal head of the big-toe joint. It can be caused by a forefoot valgus deformity that exposes the sesamoids, and/or by a type of activity that places extra pressure on the area, or by trauma. For example, a person who plays a racquet sport that requires a lot of stop-and-start running and excess pressure at a given moment on a specific part of the foot, or a woman who wears high-heeled shoes that put extra pressure on the first *metatarso-phalangeal joint* (M.P.J.) and the sesamoid bones beneath it, could be irritating the sesamoids if he or she had a forefoot valgus deformity. The inflammation can occur right under the sesamoid bone involved, or between it and the metatarsal bone above it. When the latter happens, the cartilage between the two bones becomes irritated and can degenerate to the point where bone is left rubbing against bone over a period of many years.

How do you know if you are suffering from sesamoiditis? If you have a considerable amount of pain and tenderness on the bottom of the foot under the big-toe joint when the area is palpated, you are a good candidate for sesamoiditis. The discomfort is akin to that of capsulitis or synovitis of the M.P.J., and can be exacerbated by wearing improper footwear, such as high-heeled shoes, that put undue pressure on the forefoot when the sufferer is walking. The pain may begin gradually, and might take a while to reach potentially unbearable levels. In some cases a numbing sensation may also be felt in the affected area, because of the proximity of the *proper digital nerve* that may itself become inflamed due to the irritation caused by the sesamoiditis (also Diagram 6:6). It is often difficult to determine whether the problem is one of sesamoiditis or a stress fracture of a sesamoid bone. Generally there is much more swelling if a bone is broken, and the onset of pain after the trauma causing the break is rapid and intense.

The treatment of sesamoiditis depends in large part on the cause of the disorder. If the problem originated because of a forefoot valgus deformity, the use of an orthotic device to correct the abnormality is advised. This treatment, by itself, ought to provide quick relief to the area without the need for drugs or other therapy.

If the condition resulted from a trauma, such as a sports injury, the use of ultrasound and ice ought to quiet down the area, and the inflammation will clear up on its own. If the sesamoiditis is chronic, the use of cortisone injections seems to work quite well. However, I am quite reluctant to use cortisone shots for reasons I have previously given.

Fractured Sesamoids
There are times when the sesamoids can fracture if exposed to some form of trauma or overstress. When that happens, the patient will experience pain in the area of the condition. The fracture will show up on X-rays, but there is a problem with the diagnosis nonetheless. About a fifth of all people have a *bipartite* (split in two) sesamoid bone from birth. It is a congenital condition that is harmless and painless. But when X-rays are taken of the area, it can be mistaken for a fracture of a supposedly single bone. In order to clear up the dilemma of a proper diagnosis, it may be necessary to do a bone scan of the area to determine whether or not the sesamoid has actually been fractured. The appearance of a "hot spot" on the scan will tell the tale.

Treatment of a fractured sesamoid, short of shooting the patient, is not easy. The problem is the poor supply of blood to the area, combined with the constant pounding on that part of the foot during walking or running. Once broken, a sesamoid bone will usually remain bipartite, but the pain should eventually subside and disappear.

If the pain persists to the point of affecting the patient's quality of life, a surgical approach is a definite consideration. The surgery itself involves the excision of the offending parts of the bone, but it is not a major procedure. In fact, it can be done under a local anesthetic on an out-patient basis, and the patient will be ambulatory and quite comfortable following the operation. Recovery time will depend on the patient's willingness to let the area heal naturally with as little stress as possible on it, until no discomfort is experienced during normal activities.

Here, but Forgotten
In the preceding chapters I have been discussing in great detail conditions that can affect the various parts of the foot, but I have said almost nothing—and will continue to say very little—about the

midfoot. I have been trying to figure out where I could include this boring part of the foot in the book, and I finally decided to throw in a paragraph or two at the end of this chapter so that I can get on with more exciting subject matter, but without the gnawing feeling that I have ignored something.

Look back to Diagram 2:1 to refresh your memory. It will remind you that the midfoot consists primarily of five bones: the *navicular*, three *cuneiforms*, and the *cuboid*. Obviously these bones articulate (meet to form joints) with the metatarsals and the heel bone, so that the midtarsal joint plays a role in the biomechanical function of the foot.

There is very little movement in the midtarsal joint, so the possibility of a disorder arising there is far more remote than in other parts of the foot. Also, the bones of the midfoot are very thick, almost cube-shaped, and therefore quite able to withstand punishment unless severely traumatized by some crushing accident. In my years of practice I have seen only one fractured cuboid bone, and that belonged to a weightlifter who was either careless or overly optimistic and dropped a weight on his foot.

There are certain biomechanical abnormalities that can, however, place undue stress on the midtarsal joint. As a result, some early wear-and-tear can arise and cause some mild abnormal degeneration—degeneration that could later cause osteoarthritis—but usually the condition never becomes very dramatic, and a person prone to some midfoot wear-and-tear will hardly notice any symptoms.

The midfoot can be affected by certain neuro-muscular disorders that can cause a loss of sensitivity in the area and therefore an inability to control the movement of the foot. These conditions can also cause significant degenerative changes in the midtarsal joint. However, I have seen only two people in the last ten years with such neuro-muscular diseases, so rather than worry you with details about the disorders, I would prefer to tell you that the chances of your being hit by one of them is quite remote.

Baby's Corner

Just as we have spent little time talking about the midfoot, so have we neglected the fifth, or baby, toe. Actually we did discuss the baby toe in the last chapter when we described how it can be affected by corns. The only other thing that can go wrong with it, other than being injured, is the *bunionette*—also known as a *baby bunion*, a *tailor's bunion*, or a *fifth-metatarsal-head bunion*.

These baby-toe bunions are similar to their big-toe brothers, but occur on the fifth toe rather than on the first. They are caused by two biomechanical foot faults. The first is usually congenital, and occurs when the angle between the fourth and the fifth metatarsal bones is greater than twenty per cent. Not everyone who has this abnormality will get a bunionette, but the odds increase when the angle is wider, particularly when the second biomechanical problem occurs—a plantar-flexed fifth metatarsal. In response to the extra pressure applied to the area, because the metatarsal head is never raised, the bone moves laterally away from the mid-point of the foot in an attempt to distribute the weight more evenly. Eventually a bump appears on the outside of the toe at the fifth metatarsal head in response to the irritation in the area (see Diagram 6:7). This bump corresponds to that on the big toe, but is tinier. Hence the term bunionette, or baby bunion.

DIAGRAM 6:7

The Bunionette, Its Surgical Correction, and an Avulsion Fracture

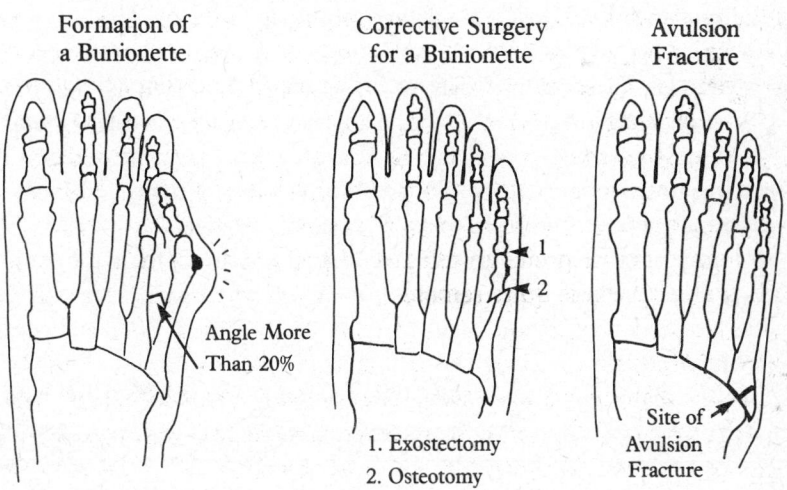

Formation of
a Bunionette

Corrective Surgery
for a Bunionette

Avulsion
Fracture

Angle More
Than 20%

1
2

1. Exostectomy
2. Osteotomy

Site of
Avulsion
Fracture

Because of the congenital nature of the problem, it is quite difficult to prevent the formation of a bunionette. Usually the only recourse is surgery once the irritation has become a real pain to the victim. The surgery involves two procedures: an *exostectomy*, or removal, of the bump on the toe, followed by an *osteotomy* to realign the metatarsal bone (also Diagram 6:7). About ninety-nine per cent of the time this surgery, whether done "open" or by using an M.I.S. technique, is successful, so successful that the patient's metatarsal is normal after a four-to-six-week recovery period.

As for the surgery itself, both the open and the M.I.S. procedures are quite similar. Only the size of the incision is different. Both use the same special drills with specially adapted bone burrs. The decision as to which technique to use will depend on the whim of the surgeon. Both procedures can be done on an out-patient basis, and the patient will usually be totally ambulatory following the operation.

The Fifth Metatarsal

Another area that is often overlooked in discussions of foot problems is the base of the fifth metatarsal bone (also Diagram 6:7). In cases where an individual has turned an ankle inwards (*lateral inversion*) moderately to severely, it is possible to actually have an *avulsion fracture* of the base of this bone. This occurs because of the dramatic force put on the bone, and is often overlooked by doctors examining and X-raying a suspected ankle fracture or similar type of injury.

The reason the fracture can be so easily overlooked is because of the proximity of the ankle bone to the base of the fifth metatarsal bone. Therefore, swelling in the area can be confused with a reaction to the ankle injury. So it will be necessary for the clinician to examine the area carefully to avoid making the mistake.

If X-rays do confirm the presence of a fractured fifth metatarsal bone at its base, the treatment is much the same as a stress fracture of any metatarsal bone. The break will heal by itself over a period of weeks without the foot having to be put in a cast or otherwise treated. But the victim will have to be careful during that recovery time not to place undue stress on the area.

7

Calluses and Warts

Life on the Underworld

Irritation to the bottom of the foot can result in excruciating pain because it is continuously supporting the weight of the body, and because the soles of the feet contain a large number of sensory nerves which are very close to the surface.

Because the underside of the foot is so sensitive, it is understandable why trials of endurance and pain involving feet have often been associated with a person's bravery and other admired qualities. (One example would be those people in certain societies who attempt to prove their valor by walking over a bed of hot coals, or nails, or both.) It is also true that, in this sometimes cruel world, the beating of the soles of the feet is a regularly preferred method of physical torture in some societies. The beating does not leave any lasting marks on the feet, so it is not easy to verify after the fact, but the pain is excruciating.

When Abe Lincoln complained publicly that his feet hurt, he may well have been referring to the bottoms of his feet, because that is where we generally feel the strain of a hard day the most, particularly if we have been "running around" for hours on end in less than perfectly comfortable footwear. Tired feet may cause you some dismay, but you can always soak them in a soothing tub to relieve the ache.

For those of you who disdain the mundane bath, my wine-loving patient has another remedy. To make this concoction you mix together 1½ ounces of talcum powder with a pint of strong red wine and two ounces of rum (either light or dark will do). You let the mixture of talcum powder and wine stand for two days before adding the

95

rum. Then you allow the entire brew to stand for one week before straining and applying it—four times daily. (I forgot to ask my patient if this concoction is to be taken internally or applied externally, or both, or drunk after the feet have been soaked in it.) The patient swears that it is the best thing around for the soothing of tired "dogs".

I will leave this, and other homebrew remedies, up to the imagination of the reader, since I intend to devote this chapter to problems that will not respond to simple tender, loving care. Suffice it to say that if the bottoms of your feet ache after a long day, and if you have no calluses, warts, or other problems that require expert attention, you need only rest your feet awhile or soak them in some solution or other to experience relief.

I hope by the end of this chapter you will be able to distinguish between feet that are merely tired and those that require professional attention.

The Callus vs. the Wart

This is not an introduction to a professional wrestling match between two villains. What I want to do before proceeding to the descriptions and treatments of calluses and warts is briefly to explain the difference between the two.

DIAGRAM 7:1
Areas Where Calluses and Warts Form

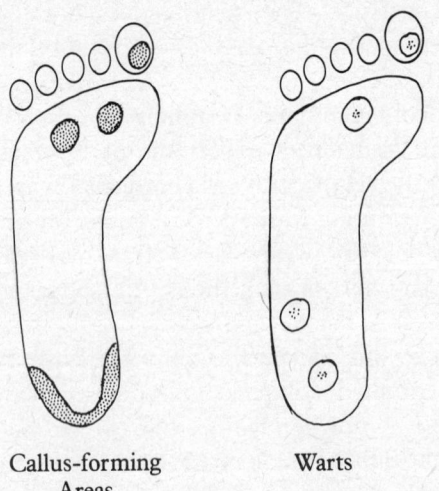

Callus-forming   Warts
Areas

As you can tell by Diagram 7:1, warts are generally quite distinct in appearance from calluses. The primary difference is the presence of blackish pin dots (*papillae*) on the warts. These dots are not found on calluses. Also, certain calluses have a whitish center core, or nucleus.

The causes of the two disorders are also as different as night and day. The wart develops after the foot has been invaded by a virus; the callus develops, like a corn, in response to pressure on an area of the bottom of the foot caused by poor weight distribution on the foot due to a biomechanical fault. As you can well imagine, treatments for the two disorders are as different as their causes.

Keep in mind, then, that the only thing a callus and a wart have in common is their location on the bottom of the foot. To the trained eye, they do not look alike. Their causes are quite different, and they are treated in totally unrelated fashions.

The Callus Truth

Calluses are often lumped together with corns in medical folklore. Like corns, they are nothing more than the build-up of thick skin to protect a part of the body that is being subjected to undue stress— in this case, the ball of the foot, which is located under the heads of the metatarsal bones. People get calluses on their hands from manual labor. However, because they do not normally walk on their hands, the calluses do not hurt unless some other forces, like squeezing a golf club, stress them. But, as mentioned, when the bottom of the foot is subjected to the pressure of body weight when a person is standing or in stride, the area where the callus has formed will hurt because ultra-sensitive sensory nerve-endings that are so close to the surface layers of the skin are irritated.

It is imperative to understand that a callus is a symptom of a disorder, not the direct cause of your discomfort. As I have mentioned, the ubiquitous biomechanical fault is usually the problem, and it can cause calluses on the bottom of the foot, particularly in areas shown in Diagram 7:1. So, while you may want to have your callus permanently and immediately removed with some magic remedy, it just is not going to happen unless the underlying cause is eliminated.

I cannot even try to count the number of times patients have asked me to get out all the roots when I am removing their calluses. There are no roots to cut out, and the calluses will reappear as long as excess pressure, caused by poor biomechanical function, is being applied to that particular area of the bottom of the foot.

The number-one enemy when it comes to the formation of calluses is abnormal pronation, which, as the foot rolls across the metatarsal heads, distributes the weight of the body unequally on the separate heads—one at a time, rather than equally. So, as you walk or run, at least one of the metatarsal heads, usually either the second or the fifth, receives the brunt of your weight with each step you take. This added stress on the burdened metatarsal head causes inflammation of the area, and a callus forms to protect the sore spot. Eventually the callus develops to the point where it becomes a problem, because the build-up of thick, dead skin, so close to the nerve endings on the underside of the foot, causes extreme pain.

One of the classic biomechanical causes of a callus is the *plantar-flexed metatarsal head*. As you will recall, in this situation one of the metatarsal heads is lower than the other four heads. What happens is that the lower-sitting head winds up absorbing as much as eighty per cent of the weight normally distributed in proper proportion across all the metatarsal heads. As a result, a severe *nucleated* callus may be formed. This type of callus has a small white center core that represents the pinpoint area of the metatarsal head where most of that excess weight is being absorbed (see Diagram 7:2). This condition is no more life-threatening than any other callus on the bottom of the foot. No matter what it may be called, or where it may develop, a callus is only thickened skin.

The position of the offending metatarsal head vis-à-vis the rest of the heads is crucial in determining the amount of build-up of callus tissue. The lower the abnormal position of the metatarsal head, the greater the development of callus tissue. If you have calluses all along the sole of your foot, it is obviously not because all the metatarsal heads are too low relative to each other. I would suspect that your troubles have a different origin, more likely a different pronation abnormality combined with a compensatory forefoot deformity. Whatever the cause of the callus growth, the primary mode of treatment is correction of the biomechanical fault causing the problem.

The metatarsal head most likely to be affected is the second (corresponding to your pointing finger), followed by the third, then the fifth. Thanks to space-age technology, the weight distribution

DIAGRAM 7:2
A Plantar-Flexed Metatarsal Head and Formation of a Nucleated Callus

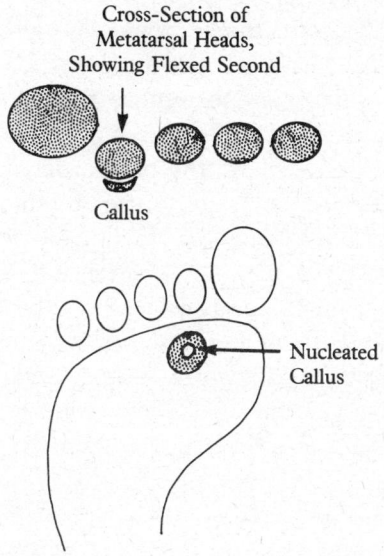

Cross-Section of
Metatarsal Heads,
Showing Flexed Second

Callus

Nucleated
Callus

on the foot when a person is in stride can be accurately computerized to determine the exact biomechanical problem, for example, the percentage of weight borne by each metatarsal head. With this information, the foot specialist can set out to normalize weight distribution on the foot during the gait cycle, and eliminate both the cause and the effect of the biomechanical fault. Of course, you already know how best to deal with the biomechanical problems that cause various foot troubles: the insertion of an orthotic device in the shoe. However, there are other treatments, depending on the severity of the condition, that can be effective. I will examine all forms of callus treatments shortly, but first I want to describe briefly remedies that ought to be avoided.

What Not To Do
Do not cut out calluses by yourself. You will suffer the same discomforts as you would with a self-excised corn. The symptoms will be relieved for a short time only, and the bathroom surgery

can lead to hospital-room treatment. Also, if any lay or professional foot specialist suggests merely removing the thickened skin without treating the underlying cause of the callus, I suggest that you seek a second opinion.

Be wary of any exotic treatments that may be presented to you as options. I have seen patients who have had a previous history of radiation treatment, surgery to remove the callus and its roots, plastic surgery to ostensibly make the area esthetically pleasing, and even partial amputation to relieve the person of the pain—and part of the foot. All of these radical options were presented to the patients without consideration being given to correcting the weight distribution that probably caused the callus in the first place.

It is more than likely that a callus will respond best to conservative, non-invasive treatment. If you are presented with a radical approach to the removal of your callus before a conservative step has been taken, run—don't walk!—as fast as you can to another doctor, preferably one who specializes in feet.

The Right Step

Now that you know what not to do when you have a bothersome callus, you are ready for the next step—and the right step.

Our old friend the orthotic device again comes to the rescue. The orthotic works to eliminate the weight-distribution problem on the metatarsal heads, whether that condition is due to a plantar-flexed metatarsal head or to another biomechanical dysfunction, or to a combination of disorders. Not only does the device correct the weight-distribution discrepancy if it is properly fitted, it also serves to raise a low metatarsal head. Once the biomechanical fault has been eliminated, an ordinary callus will disappear slowly by itself—over a six-to-twelve-month period.

A nucleated callus, however, requires treatment on a regular basis every few weeks, even after the biomechanical cause has been eliminated with the use of an orthotic. This is because old habits are often hard to break, and the foot has been tricked by habit to form callus tissue. It may continue to do so, although the irritation no longer exists. The remains of the nucleated callus should be trimmed by an expert with a sharp knife. Once again, I cannot stress too strongly how dangerous it is for you to do this at home. The risk of cutting too deep is real; the consequences are infection and other damage to healthy tissue, and the possible formation of scar tissue.

Break-lancing

If a serious callus is being caused by a severely plantar-flexed metatarsal head, and if your quality of life is being adversely affected by the discomfort, surgery may be required to correct the malformation of the bone, because the problem cannot be eliminated by wearing an orthotic device.

As with much foot surgery, the correction of a plantar-flexed metatarsal head can be done using either an "open" or a "closed" (M.I.S.) osteotomy procedure. Both can be performed in a doctor's office under local anesthetic. In either case, the risk of infection is minimal, and the patient is ambulatory immediately after the operation. However, there appears to be less discomfort with the M.I.S. technique, since the incision is smaller and there is less overall trauma to the area.

The success rate for plantar-flexed-metatarsal-head surgery is about eighty per cent. In the twenty per cent that fail, the problem is usually that the bone has been raised too high relative to the position of the adjacent metatarsal bones. You can guess what happens in that situation. You wind up with one or two metatarsal heads, adjacent to the one that was operated on, that are now too low relative to the others on the foot, and on the bottom of the foot under these newly affected metatarsal heads you will soon discover the development of calluses to protect the area from the stress of a weight load that is too heavy. You may have traded in a callus in one area for another in a different area.

How long does it take the foot to heal after a successful osteotomy? Rest assured that if you ever do require such surgery, you should be able to walk out of the doctor's office unaided, with minimal discomfort, immediately after the procedure—whether it is "open" or "closed". The doctor will explain to you how to keep the area bandaged, how to cleanse the wound from the incision, and what activities to avoid, and for how long. Providing that you take it easy— in other words, avoid running marathons or engaging in other strenuous physical activities until the area has healed—you should completely heal within six to twelve weeks. And, assuming that the operation was a success, the callus should have disappeared in three to six months.

Sometimes a biomechanical fault can cause nucleated calluses under two or more metatarsal heads at one time. When that happens, surgical intervention (an osteotomy) will be required. While an orthotic may work well if only one or two bones are involved, it is much more difficult if more than two metatarsals are affected, because it is then much harder to equalize weight distribution. There are simply too many abnormal metatarsal heads that require equalizing. If orthotics fail to provide relief, all the abnormal metatarsal heads may have to be surgically corrected to restore weight-distribution balance to the foot.

You may think by now that calluses occur only under the front part, or ball, of the foot. The truth is that they are indeed most often found there, but they do occur, though less frequently, on the heel of the foot. So, before we tackle warts, we ought to take the time to discuss callused heels.

The Callused Heel
The callused heel is a foot doctor's nemesis, because it is not easy to treat successfully. Actually the calluses form around the edges of the heel, and rarely on the bottom. If you do discover something unusual on the bottom of your heel, it is most likely a wart, and not a callus.

Unlike calluses under the metatarsal heads on the soles of your feet, calluses on the edges of the heel are not caused by a weight-distribution problem. They are the result of the combined effects of dry skin and constant irritation caused by a particular shoe. Since I intend to discuss skin problems of the foot in a later chapter, I will not go into great detail here about the treatment of skin conditions. However, I will tell you that orthotic devices to treat heel calluses will be useless, since the problem is not biomechanical. In fact, the device may itself increase the irritation around the heel callus, thereby aggravating the problem. Also mere trimming of the callus will provide relief for only a few weeks.

In more obstreperous cases, heel calluses can become so dry and hard that they crack. This results in a *fissure (lesion)* of the skin, and the area may bleed and become infected. If the fissuring is mild, apply a good commercial moisturizing cream to the affected area and then cover it with a plastic film wrapping, such as Saran Wrap, to hold in the body's moisture. Leave the application on through the night, shower in the morning, and then use a pumice stone to smooth the callused area. With luck, you will experience relief in a few weeks.

If the condition is more severe, you will probably have to visit a foot doctor in order to prevent the breaking down, the cracking, and the possible development of an infection at the site. But, once the callused area has begun to improve, with the help of antibiotic cream, soaking, and the use of a pumice stone, the doctor will more than likely tell you to revert to the daily application of moisturizing creams at home. If the problem is particularly difficult, and a serious infection develops, it may be necessary to take antibiotics orally.

In general, callused heels are not miraculously cured overnight. Constant care and patience are the two ingredients required to treat the condition. Anyone who has suffered through a lifetime of dry skin will understand the difficulty. So far, medical researchers have failed to develop a panacea for many dermatological disorders, and dry skin anywhere on the body is no exception. As far as heel calluses are concerned, however, there is one thing a person can do to improve the situation, and that is to wear more comfortable shoes that do not irritate the sides of your heels.

Warts and All
There are two different types of warts found on the bottom of the foot, and less commonly elsewhere on the foot. Both of them are caused by the *papilloma virus*. The most common of these is the *verruca vulgaris*—a combination of Latin and medicalese for "the common wart". The verruca vulgaris accounts for about ninety-five per cent of all warts on the bottom of the foot, and occurs singly most of the time, although it can occasionally occur in clusters of five or six (see Diagram 7:3).

The other type of wart is called a *mosaic verruca* because of its mosaic appearance (also Diagram 7:3). It usually occurs in clusters of fifty to sixty little growths in one concentrated area. Although it has not been scientifically proved, I suspect that the mosaic verruca

DIAGRAM 7:3
Two Kinds of Wart

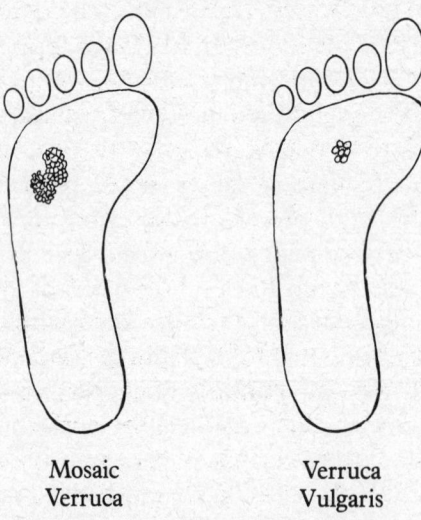

Mosaic
Verruca

Verruca
Vulgaris

is caused by an offshoot of the verruca vulgaris. The mosaic wart is far more difficult to treat than the common wart because the virus is much more widespread in the area, and is not easily totally destroyed.

A Viral Attack

Contrary to popular fairy tales, warts are not caused by an intimate encounter with a toad, a curse from a witch, or abnormal behavior. The papilloma virus is solely to blame. This little devil, like all of its cousins in the virus mafia, flourishes in all sorts of environments and can be picked up and transmitted by humans when the proper conditions exist. When the virus invades the bottom of the foot, a *plantar* wart will develop. It is called a "plantar" wart because it grows on the bottom, or "plantar", part of the foot, not because it grows like some plant or is well-planted with roots under the skin.

Although it has yet to be medically proven, I believe that there must be a readily available blood supply to a particular area to allow the wart to begin growing. So, while the papilloma virus may indeed be contagious, it is so only when the proper conditions exist for it to find a new home. For a plantar wart to develop, the virus must enter the bottom of the foot through an abrasion or puncture wound, and there must be a good supply of blood to the site. There are two other factors that contribute to the successful invasion of the virus. First, it requires warmth as well as nourishment to flourish. The bottom of the foot usually meets that requirement. Second, the virus has to outfox the body's natural immunological system. Most experts and plantar-wart sufferers will agree that the warts are very difficult to treat, because viruses in general have been able to outsmart the natural defences of many people, and the research of medical scientists. Mankind is still waiting for a cure or prevention for the common cold, which is caused by a host of viral infections.

Once the virus that causes the plantar wart establishes a foothold, it spreads and multiplies to form a painful growth. It hurts so much because it usually finds a weight-bearing part of the foot to nest in. The tiny black dots that form on the surface of the wart are nothing more than tiny blood vessels that nourish it. Many people who look at these discolorations automatically assume that they are the ends of the roots of the wart. This is pure nonsense; warts no more have roots than do corns and calluses.

The papilloma virus is also very clever when it comes to self-preservation. It outsmarts the efforts of the body's natural defences by forming a capsule around the developing wart. This encapsulation prevents the body's immune system from attacking and killing off the virus. However, the virus is quite content to remain in the superficial layers of the skin, so the wart does not penetrate very far below the surface of its host. But, because the virus is so clever, it may somehow hide itself under the skin, even though the wart itself has been totally removed. This is why the wart itself could return in the very same spot where it originally developed.

Wart Removal
The best way to deal with plantar warts is to try and prevent them from developing in the first place. Since the virus will enter the skin through a wound of some kind, the logical solution is to ensure that no lesion in the skin ever occurs. Of course, that is not always possible.

Because of some of the reasons I have mentioned, once the virus has penetrated the skin on the bottom of the foot, it will be difficult to dislodge. Some viruses, including the papilloma variety, are like unwanted house guests that hang around under foot until the host finally gathers together his or her resources to strike back and force the unwelcome intruders to leave. During that time, however, the intruders can create a fair amount of discomfort, and may eventually have to be physically removed with harsh measures. And they may return.

Naturally, you do not want to burn down the house to get rid of your unwanted guests, unless you need the insurance money. Neither do you want to destroy healthy body tissue on the bottom of your foot to get rid of a plantar wart. Keep this in mind as we discuss the various treatments. It is also important to consider that warts in general have a life span of about two years—although I have known some to hang around longer. Therefore, if you are not unduly distressed by the presence of a wart on your foot, or elsewhere, you might decide to let nature take its course.

Potatoes, Cod-Liver Oil, and Other Snake-Oil Remedies

There are so many old wives' tales, and new theories, when it comes to the treatment of plantar warts, that they are almost impossible to catalogue. What amazes me is that so many of them occasionally seem to work, despite medical logic. It is downright embarrassing to the medical profession. My rule of thumb when dealing with plantar warts has become that if the cure is not potentially worse than the disease, by all means try it.

One such cure was brought to my attention recently by a woman patient I had unsuccessfully treated for a plantar wart for over two years. I had tried all the conventional methods—surgery, acids, liquid nitrogen, and a host of different creams—with no lasting success. The woman was in considerable discomfort, because the wart was strategically located on the ball of her foot—a prime weight-bearing area.

One day, her eighty-seven-year-old next-door neighbor told her to rub the wart with a potato, and then store the potato in a kitchen cupboard for one month. My patient did so, and thirty days later the wart was gone. It has not returned. As a last resort, I now suggest to my patients with stubborn plantar warts that they try the same method.

One of my patients tried various home and medical remedies before he got rid of his plantar wart with hypnosis therapy. It is apparently true that warts are susceptible to the power of suggestion. So it would seem logical that hypnotic suggestion would work if the hypothesis is true. It may also explain why potatoes or spitting saliva on a wart will make it go away. If you believe strongly in these fairy-tale cures, they may well be successful. My studies have shown me that psychosomatic treatment combined with more conventional treatment methods seems to work better than on its own. But the definitive word has yet to be spoken.

If potatoes, saliva, or hypnosis fail to work, there are other folklorish remedies to consider. One old remedy is to be found in an old English textbook on dermatology. The treatment entails the external application four or five times daily, via a cotton swab, of cod-liver oil. I was curious about this method, and decided to try it for the first time on a nineteen-year-old female diabetic patient for whom I had exhausted all other forms of non-surgical therapy. Because of her diabetes she was a poor risk for surgery.

Lo and behold, after about five weeks of cod-liver-oil applications to the area, the plantar wart disappeared entirely. I was impressed. I subsequently discovered that cod-liver oil enhanced with vitamin A has proved to be almost ninety per cent effective in the removal of plantar warts, at least according to my experience and research. However, the treatment does not provide an overnight cure, so the patient must have patience.

A few months ago I was on a radio talk show and I mentioned this cure for plantar warts in response to a question by a listener. Within a few weeks I had received numerous testimonials in the mail attesting to the fact that the cod-liver-oil treatment really works.

I wish I knew why cod-liver oil seems to destroy the papilloma virus, but I do not. I have asked various virologists and other medical researchers, and the general conclusion is that perhaps the high content of vitamin A in the oil has something to do with its viral-fighting qualities.

I am sure there are many other harmless treatments, old and new, available for plantar and other warts. If I wanted to devote an entire chapter—even a book—to such remedies, I am certain that I would have no trouble doing so. But I want now to examine other ways of removing plantar warts for good.

Acids

There are also numerous acid products sold over the counter in drug stores for the treatment of warts; and there are more potent acids used by doctors that are not readily available to the public. These solutions are generally effective in about only sixty per cent of the cases. This percentage may be slightly higher, since doctors usually see only those people who have failed to gain relief from the over-the-counter preparations.

The acid that a doctor will use is a sixty-per-cent-salicylic-acid solution that is available in either a cream or on medicated pads. This acid is applied twice daily. After showering, you smooth the warty area with a pumice stone to remove layers of the wart. Eventually, the bottom of the wart will be reached. Once again, if you happen to carry a rabbit's foot, you may be lucky enough to kill the papilloma virus completely by removing all the layers, and the wart will never return.

There are also acid-plaster dressings that can be applied weekly to a wart. And once a week the wart is peeled off layer by layer, until no friendly environment exists in which the virus can thrive. Unfortunately, this works only about fifty to sixty per cent of the time. The virus is very adaptable, even in hostile environments.

One problem with the use of over-the-counter or prescription acid treatments is the temptation to abuse the solution. If one drop is good, two ought to be better and quicker, and ten ought to be fantastic. Of course, what happens with an over-application of an acid is a nasty acid burn. Also, without medical direction, you might be using an over-the-counter preparation for warts when the problem is actually a callus that has to be treated as a biomechanical dysfunction of the foot. Warts treated as calluses, on the other hand, rarely respond positively, unless a callus has developed around the wart to protect the area of the bottom of the foot from the painful pressure of the wart. In that case, the treatment indicated is twofold: biomechanical correction for the callus, and topical medication for the wart.

Freeze!

Liquid nitrogen works a little like a laser beam and an acid. Because it is at such a low temperature (-276°C) when it is applied to a wart, it freezes (or burns, or vaporizes) the growth, which then blisters and can be peeled away in layers until only the bottom layer remains. A final application of the liquid nitrogen then removes the last of the wart and, hopefully, the rest of the papilloma virus. Sad to say, this treatment works in only about sixty per cent of the cases on which it is tried.

Surgery

If all of the above methods for the non-surgical removal of a plantar wart have failed, and if the patient is suffering from an unacceptable level of discomfort and dysfunction, it may be necessary to resort to an excision procedure. I want to emphasize, however, that surgery is often no more effective than any of the non-invasive treatments, and could leave the patient with even more discomfort than he/she began with. That is because scar tissue may form where the skin has been cut, and that scarring can be very painful, since the patient will be walking and putting pressure on the area constantly. Another problem with surgery is that it can cause problems in patients who suffer from circulatory and/or other systemic disorders. Healing will be much slower, and the risk of post-operative infection far greater, than in normal, healthy patients. Actually, I try to avoid operating on the bottom of the foot, whatever the problem, unless I have absolutely no choice.

Shedding Light on Laser Surgery

The Pentagon does not have a monopoly on enthusiasm when it comes to laser beams. Laser surgery is making quantum leaps, and I suspect that in the near future it will replace much of what is now the state-of-the-art in the operating room. As I have mentioned, there is also much room for the use of lasers to treat foot problems that might normally require invasive procedures.

Podiatrists have now begun using laser beams to vaporize warts. In the last few years they have achieved over a ninety-five-per-cent success rate. The beauty of laser surgery on the bottom of the foot is that the problem of scarring is basically eliminated because the tissue under the wart is not damaged in the process. The major obstacle to the common use of laser surgery by podiatrists is the high cost of the equipment. At present, the laser equipment I would like to purchase for my office costs about $50,000. No doubt the price will drop, as did the price of computers, once the equipment becomes widely used.

Wrapping Up the Wart

By now you may have decided what you are going to do if you are unlucky enough to develop a plantar wart, or a wart on any other part of the body for that matter. You may have also realized that there is no one-hundred-per-cent solution to the problem.

There is another option, as I mentioned earlier in the chapter. Most warts will go away by themselves—eventually. Some disappear without any treatment whatsoever in a matter of weeks, while others will hang around for years. If you are a patient person who is not in any considerable discomfort from a plantar wart, I suggest again that you simply try to wait it out.

One step I strongly urge you *not* to take is to try and cut out the wart by yourself. You could cause yourself a lot of grief by cutting too deep, and thereby creating an extensive amount of scar tissue, and/or setting yourself up for a nasty infection. As I mentioned in earlier chapters, I strongly urge people to avoid bathroom surgery at all costs.

Finally, I want to remind you again that whatever steps you take, make sure that you know what it is that you have on the bottom of your foot—a callus or a wart. If you fail to diagnose the disorder properly, your efforts to eliminate the problem yourself will be for naught.

8
Down at the Heels: Disorders of the Rearfoot

Somehow over the years the poor downtrodden heel has acquired a bad reputation. In American jargon a heel is a despicable person who has a shocking lack of decency or honor. And, going all the way back to Greek mythology, another rear portion of the foot—the Achilles tendon—has become synonymous with weakness. Nothing could be farther from the truth. In fact, the heel is a very useful part of the human anatomy and there is no reason whatsoever to associate it with lowlife. The heel has tremendous shock-absorbing qualities that protect the rest of the body from undue stress, and is most important to one's gait. When you consider the constant pounding to which it is subjected, often on hard, uneven surfaces, over many, many years, it is amazing that the heel remains as healthy as it does.

However, if the rearfoot is injured in any way, it is often slower to heal (no pun intended) than other parts of the body, because of the poor supply of blood to the area. For example, tendons will normally heal by themselves if ruptured (torn). But the Achilles tendon will often have to be surgically repaired because of the lack of fresh, healing nutrients that reach its cells. And fractures of the bones in the back of the foot will also take longer to heal—and will be quite painful longer—for the same reason. Fortunately, fractures of the bones in the rearfoot are rare, for reasons I will describe below.

As with other parts of the foot, there are quite a few myths floating around concerning the heel and what can go wrong with it and with adjacent parts of the lower limbs. (Incidentally, very little will be said in this chapter about the ankle, since this joint is very sturdy and well-designed. Ankle problems are usually traumatically induced, and, for that reason, they will be discussed primarily in the chapters on sports medicine.) A lot of these old stories are now coming under closer scrutiny, as running has become more and more popular, and athletes are succumbing to abnormalities of the rearfoot. In fact, I see quite a few cases of heel- and ankle-area injuries weekly at the Mount Sinai Hospital S.C. Cooper Family Sports Medicine Clinic. In a good number of these cases, the patient has no concept of what the problem really is. Actually, such patients are not alone; there are many medical professionals who also have trouble diagnosing conditions affecting the rearfoot.

There are numerous reasons for pain in the rearfoot, and in this chapter I intend to discuss the most common: *plantar fasciitis*, *Achilles tendonitis*, *Haglund's deformity*, and the *tarsal-tunnel syndrome*. There are a few unusual disorders I have omitted because they are rare, and of a complexity that requires explanations that would require a medical textbook full of terrible medicalese.

Let us examine the rearfoot to learn what exactly can go wrong. As you can see in Diagram 8:1, the two major bones at the rear of the foot are the ankle bone (*talus*) and the heel bone (*calcaneus*). Together with other bones in the area they help form the *tarsus*— the rear part of the foot, including the ankle. When we have a sore heel, we most often blame it on a problem with the heel bone, but that is usually a mis-diagnosis, because the actual cause of the discomfort is not from a bruise or a break in the bone, but from the inflammation of the adjoining soft tissue.

DIAGRAM 8:1
The Two Major Bones of the Heel

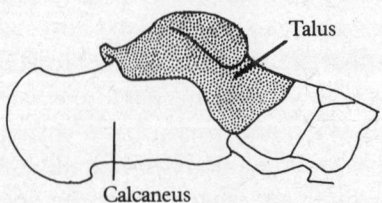

Talus

Calcaneus

Before we get to the inflammation of the soft tissues, we ought to examine the heel bone—to understand why it is so difficult to seriously injure. As you can see from Diagram 8:2, the heel bone is a solid, block-like structure, well protected by soft tissue which surrounds it and acts like a cushion. It can be broken or bruised, but only by a traumatic, concussive injury, such as a fall from higher than twenty feet.

DIAGRAM 8:2
The Well-Protected Heel Bone

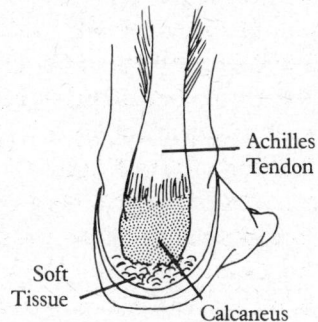

Achilles
Tendon

Soft
Tissue

Calcaneus

In all my years of practicing podiatry, I have only twice seen a fractured heel bone. In the first instance a Hydro worker fell forty feet onto concrete pavement, and landed heels first. I am sure he was much happier to have landed feet first rather than head first; a fractured heel bone will heal faster than a fractured skull, and will generally have far fewer side effects—if the person survives the fall.

The second case was not quite as serious, and involved a rather comic but potentially tragic incident. I was summoned to the emergency room of the hospital I work out of one evening to examine the foot of a middle-aged man who had been forced to make a hasty retreat from the bedroom of his mistress, when her husband returned from a trip much earlier than anticipated. The man had jumped out of the third-floor bedroom window, and had been lucky enough to land feet first on the ground. He was so frightened that he ran for almost a mile before he realized that he had sustained a serious injury to the heel of one foot. I am sure that, considering the circumstances, he was quite relieved to escape with just a fractured heel bone.

Breaching the Heel

If the heel bone rarely fractures or bruises, what then is the cause of heel pain? As I have already mentioned, in order to understand the cause of the discomfort, we have to look to the soft tissue in the area, particularly the *plantar fascia* and the *Achilles tendon*.

As you can see from Diagram 8:3, the heel bone is affected by the Achilles tendon, which is attached at the rear of the bone, and by the plantar fasciae, which are connected to the bottom front part of the bone. In a sense, the tendon and the fasciae compete with each other to influence the actions of the heel bone when a person is walking or running. When an abnormality occurs because one of these soft-tissue masses forces the other to overstress—for a variety of reasons, including poor biomechanics of the lower limbs—rearfoot pain occurs due to the resulting inflammation. The sufferer often believes this pain to be from the heel bone.

DIAGRAM 8:3
Heel-Bone Attachments

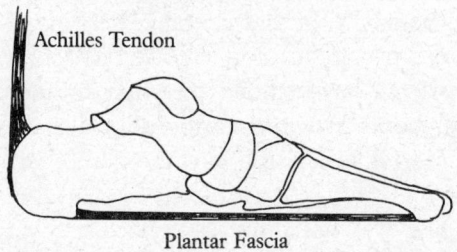

Achilles Tendon

Plantar Fascia

Because the plantar fasciae and the Achilles tendon pull in 90-degree opposing directions, it is not uncommon for both of them to become inflamed almost simultaneously, causing *Achilles tendonitis* (inflammation of the Achilles tendon) and *plantar fasciitis* (inflammation of the plantar fasciae). These two conditions are the main causes of rearfoot pain, so let us look at them in greater detail.

Plantar Fasciitis

Athletes, particularly runners, are well aware of the problem of plantar fasciitis, but, as is the case with the general public, they do not really understand the disorder, and they are saddled with numerous myths about how it is caused and how it ought to be treated. Well, even medical professionals are in difficulty when it comes to plantar fasciitis, specially when they have yet to agree as to whether the plantar fascia is a tendon or a ligament.

As you can see in Diagram 8:4, the plantar fasciae are attached to the heel bone and to the five metatarsal bones that are situated in the forefoot. The fasciae have two tasks to perform: the first is to support the longitudinal arch of the foot, and the second is to help prevent over-pronation.

DIAGRAM 8:4
Heel-Spur Development and the Site of Fascia Tearing

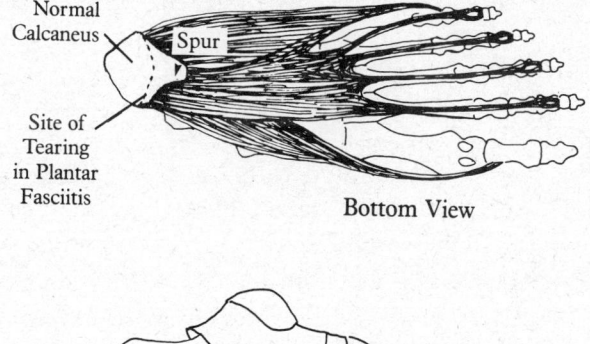

Normal Calcaneus

Spur

Site of Tearing in Plantar Fasciitis

Bottom View

Normal Calcaneus with Spur Formation

Spur

Side View

If the subtalar joint is abnormally pronating, the plantar fasciae, which are already tightly strung in their normal condition, become stretched even further as they try to prevent the abnormal pronation from occurring. This extra stress on the fasciae can eventually cause them to become inflamed and to tear away from their attachment at the heel bone (also Diagram 8:4). When this happens, plantar fasciitis develops, and the area becomes quite uncomfortable. If you can imagine pulling a tuft of hair from your head, you will have a fair analogy to the discomfort of plantar fasciitis.

While the plantar fascia fibers are often torn away from the heel bone in trying to prevent the foot from over-pronating, abnormal pronation is not the sole cause of plantar fasciitis. In the high-arched, semi-flexible or rigid foot, there is added pressure on the plantar fasciae to prevent biomechanical problems associated with such conditions from occurring. Also, it appears that, in older people, the plantar fasciae tend to lose much of their elasticity, thereby causing excessive strain to the area where the fasciae connect to the heel bone. As you may expect, plantar fasciitis then occurs as the area becomes inflamed.

Plantar fasciitis can plague its victims for years. I have one patient who has suffered from the disorder for twelve years, during which time he has had a total of four operations to try and correct the problem. The surgery involved is quite controversial and rarely warranted. This particular patient is now feeling much better, but he still has occasional recurrences of the disorder.

Spurring the Truth

Plantar fasciitis is often confused with *heel spurs*. I have lost count of the number of people who have told me that they suffer from heel spurs because they were told so by another doctor, or by a friend with a similar problem. But people do not *suffer* from heel spurs, because heel spurs do not cause pain. They develop in response to a painful situation, in an attempt to relieve the discomfort.

Heel spurs are not really spurs at all. They are ridges when seen head on, although they may look like spurs in a two-dimensional X-ray. Regardless of their actual appearance, their development can be explained by a simple theory of kinestheology—bone conforms to stress under which it has been placed.

When a situation occurs that causes the plantar fasciae to pull hard at the area where they are attached to the heel bone, that bone eventually begins to grow in the direction of the pull. This is nature's way of shortening the extension of the plantar fasciae to relieve the excess pressure on them. All things being equal, the inflammation around the stressed area will then heal. Unfortunately, however, this is not always the case.

But, in any event, it is the soft tissue itself that hurts, not the bone, because the bone has no nerve endings there. If surgery is undertaken to relieve plantar fasciitis pain, it is soft tissue that is cut away from the bone; the bone itself is usually left untouched. Studies have shown that if both feet have heel spurs, the pain is almost negligible where the ridge is longer. In fact, should the heel ridge grow sufficiently, the pain from the plantar fasciitis would disappear totally.

So, in summation, a heel spur grows in response to the long-term existence of plantar fasciitis, since such a chronic inflammatory process at the attachment of the plantar fasciae to the heel bone creates *osteoblastic activity* (new bone growth). People do not *suffer* from heel spurs; the heel-bone shape changes to counter the causes and effects of plantar fasciitis.

Oh, How I Hate To Get Up in the Morning!
The classic characteristic of plantar fasciitis is pain in the area of the inflammation when pressure is first put on the foot in the morning. Once a person with the disorder has been walking around for a few minutes, the pain subsides, and the normal daily routine can be conducted without too much discomfort in the heel area. However, any lengthy time spent sitting or lying during the day will bring on the pain, as soon as weight is again put on the foot. The sufferer will most likely believe that the pain is caused by a bone bruise, but the bone involved—the heel bone—is not easy to injure, as we have already learned. The culprit is the plantar fascia.

There are two schools of thought as to why the area is so sore after a person has been off his or her feet for a long period of time and then puts weight on the affected foot. Some experts believe that the fasciae try to heal themselves whenever the foot is not on the ground. This healing process is rudely interrupted when the person stands on the foot, and puts weight on the offending area. Renewed tearing of the fasciae takes place, and the pain becomes severe. However, if this theory were completely valid, why then does the pain subside to tolerable levels after a few minutes of walking?

The second theory, to which I subscribe more readily, is that the plantar fasciae contract during the night, when the feet are being totally rested, and are therefore very tight and sore when they are first subjected to weight-bearing in the morning. As they naturally stretch out, the plantar fasciae become less stressed, and the pain subsides as the person continues to walk. This would seem to be the more plausible explanation, considering that the pain does subside after a few minutes of walking.

Becoming Well-Heeled: Part I

The successful treatment of plantar fasciitis is a double-barrelled endeavor. On one hand, the inflammation must be dealt with; on the other, the cause of the disorder must be eliminated. In mild cases, the elimination of the cause will also eliminate the need for treatment of the inflammation itself. When the inflammation is more severe, it will have to be attacked more vigorously.

It has been accepted practice for years to treat painful plantar fasciitis inflammations with injections of cortisone and a local anesthetic. The procedure often provides immediate relief that can last for six to twelve weeks, but the disorder will return because the cause of the problem will not have been eliminated. I have injected less than five per cent of my patients, because cortisone shots have side effects, as I have already mentioned. It is also fairly common today to prescribe anti-inflammatory drugs, other than cortisone or similar steroids, that are taken orally. However, all anti-inflammatory drugs have some potential side effects that may outweigh the benefits in the long run. Moreover, no anti-inflammatory drug that I know of will prevent abnormal pronation by itself.

If plantar fasciitis is caused by a traumatic injury to the foot, the use of an anti-inflammatory drug may clear up the condition by itself, since there is no underlying biomechanical fault in the foot.

In many cases, where the use of an anti-inflammatory drug is not indicated, physiotherapy may help somewhat. Ultrasound is the treatment most often recommended. Icing down the area may also help relieve the inflammation. However, physiotherapy on its own will not normally cure the condition. In cases where a biomechanical fault does not necessitate the use of a special orthotic device, a simple, inexpensive arch-support may make walking more bearable during the recovery stage.

In most cases of plantar fasciitis, however, the culprit is over-pronation, and the treatment is a custom-made orthotic device. Keep in mind, however, that the device only prevents the development of the condition; it does not relieve an inflammation that is severe enough to require pain-killing treatment. The reason that the orthotic device provides permanent long-term relief is that it eliminates the excessive pull on the plantar fasciae by preventing over-pronation of the foot. When the foot no longer over-pronates, there is no need for the plantar fasciae to over-extend themselves to the point where they may tear away from the heel bone. It has been my experience that ninety per cent of plantar fasciitis cases are successfully treated by the fitting of proper orthotics. Even in many severe, chronic cases, when over-pronation has been excessive, an insert by itself has done the trick, and the heel has healed without the need for drugs or physiotherapy.

It must be stressed, however, that orthotics do not provide immediate relief. It takes time for the plantar fasciae to heal and to return to their normal condition. So you will have to be patient; eventually your heel will probably feel as good as new—if not better.

Occasionally an injury will occur that requires a different form of treatment. In my capacity as team podiatrist for the Toronto Blue Jays baseball team, I have treated more than one ball-player who has twisted a foot by taking a bad step on a base and has stretched the plantar fasciae. The treatment in such cases requires the application of a "longitudinal and metatarsal" pad which is held in place by a "low dye" strapping (see Diagram 8:5). The padding and taping take the stress off the plantar fasciae and enable the area to heal fairly quickly. One player I treated this way returned to action in three days.

Other athletes, and active people in general, are often hampered by soreness in the back part of their feet, and they resort to various types of heel cushions to protect themselves from their imaginary heel-spur disease. These foamy cushions are a regular feature in my office, since most patients I see with plantar fasciitis wear them in

DIAGRAM 8:5
Low-Dye Strapping

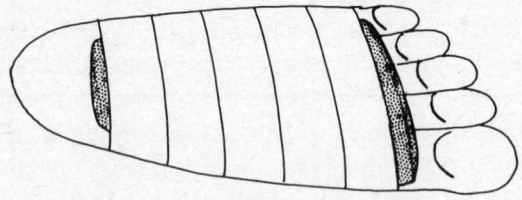

Quarter-Inch Felt Pad with Four to
Five Two-Inch Tape Strips

their shoes constantly in the mistaken belief that they will give them relief. Well, if they did work, why are all these people in my waiting room?

The reason the heel cushions do not work for plantar fasciitis is that they do nothing to prevent over-pronation. I suggest to my patients that they save their money to buy an inexpensive pair of properly constructed, perfectly fitting running-shoes that will have a proper arch-support and perhaps an anti-roll bar (not the kind found in racing cars) that acts to prevent over-pronation. These shoes will not provide a one-hundred-per-cent cure for plantar fasciitis, but they will help in many instances.

One of the stranger foam-padded cushions I have seen has its middle cut out, donut shape, to protect the "painful" heel spur. Actually, the cushion is quite useless from that point of view, and has absolutely no effect on the ridge of bone, but it does accidentally help the plantar fasciae by supporting them at the front, and alleviating their over-stretching. In fact, if you were to combine the donut-shaped pad with a decent arch-support, you would wind up with the optimal piecemeal treatment. Now, whoever said that the hole in the donut was useless?

Only one of my plantar fasciitis patients has required surgery, and he had suffered from the disorder for twenty-three years. His condition was exacerbated by an occupational hazard: he was a Hydro worker who was constantly climbing up Hydro poles and positioning his feet awkwardly to avoid losing his grip. (Incidentally, he was not the same fellow who fell off a Hydro pole and fractured his heel bone.)

There are two distinct surgical procedures for plantar fasciitis, both of which are done using M.I.S. techniques. The fact that the patient may have heel spurs at the same time plays no role in either procedure. Since I do not believe in operating for plantar fasciitis, except in very rare cases, I will not discuss these techniques further.

The Achilles Heel

Just in case you don't know how the tendon that attaches at the heel bone and runs up the bottom of the leg to the calf got its name, here is the story as it has been handed down throughout the ages, as part of Greek mythology.

Achilles was a Greek king of great acclaim as a warrior and healer. It was told that when he was a child, his mother, Thetis, took him by one heel and dipped him in the river Styx to make him physically invulnerable. But, unfortunately for the poor lad, the heel held in his mother's hand remained dry, and was therefore vulnerable. Eventually he was slain by Paris—according to some Greek mythological poems—who fired an arrow into Achilles' heel, the one weak spot on his body. (Occasionally when I think of that story, I wonder what might have happened to lay medical terminology and certain common phrases had Achilles' mother held him by another appendage.)

When medical professionals speak of Achilles, they refer not to the heel itself, but to the tendon that is a vital part of the rearfoot. We also tend to mutter obscenities under our breath when we run across a case of Achilles tendonitis—an inflammation of the Achilles tendon. Achilles tendonitis is difficult to treat, particularly when one is dealing with an athlete who wants to rush back to his/her activity long before the inflammation has cleared up, and who might be willing to risk a recurrence of the problem on a regular basis in order to indulge in a favorite pastime.

However, it is not always the dedicated athlete that we see with Achilles tendonitis. The most common victims, in fact, are women between the ages of twenty and forty-five. Let me explain why these women are so prone to the disorder.

Some women begin wearing shoes with a heel height of from two to four inches when they are still growing teenagers. They continue to wear high-heeled pumps as they enter the white-collar work force, because they do not want to look out of place in the office. As the years go by, these young women develop shortened Achilles tendons, because the tendon no longer has to stretch down to enable the foot to sit comfortably in a regular-heeled shoe. As a urologist colleague of mine once said, "If you don't use it, it shrivels up."

Now, what happens when a woman who has been wearing high-heeled shoes almost exclusively throughout her mature years suddenly decides to become natural and/or athletic and change into low-heeled shoes for running, walking, or other activities? If her Achilles tendon has shortened substantially, she will not have the tendon length required to allow her foot to sit properly in the low-heeled shoe. The tendon then tries to stretch to reach down to the back of the foot, which is now positioned differently in relation to the lower leg. We saw what happens to the plantar fasciae when they are over-stretched. The same happens to the Achilles tendon: it becomes inflamed, and tendonitis develops (see Diagram 8:6). Unless the problem is corrected, the condition will become chronic, particularly during the summer months when the woman may be wearing low-heeled shoes more often, and switching back and forth between high and low heels regularly. As long as the woman continues to wear high-heeled shoes exclusively, she will avoid the tendonitis. Of course, as you already know, high-heeled shoes cause a host of other foot problems.

(Incidentally, men who have worn two-inch-heel boots their entire adult life, and then begin exercising in one-inch-heel running-shoes, may also develop an Achilles-tendon problem.)

The next most common cause of Achilles tendonitis—a cause that affects both male and female—is congenital. Some babies are born with Achilles tendons that are too short, and they stay that way unless the situation is alleviated either by a program of stretching exercises, or by surgery to lengthen the tendon. If you see tots who walk exclusively on their toes, it is quite likely that their Achilles tendons are too short. Tiptoeing in this case has nothing to do with stealth or speed.

The third most common cause of Achilles tendonitis is overstress of the tendon and the area surrounding it. This most often affects athletes, and is a classic "overuse" syndrome. The irritation to the tendon produces an inflammation that tends to become chronic because the athlete does not rest or treat the traumatized area sufficiently. The condition is often exacerbated by a biomechanical fault, particularly abnormal pronation, that is ignored until the inflammation becomes quite severe. And, occasionally, the injury to the Achilles tendon is made worse by some traumatic episode, such as the sufferer taking a bad step and "turning" the ankle. Of course, such an occurrence can also strike the non-athlete, who may slip on a stair and have one foot land awkwardly on a step below, badly pulling the Achilles tendon.

Before I discuss treatment techniques for Achilles tendonitis, I want to define more precisely exactly what the disorder involves. As I mentioned above, Achilles tendonitis is an inflammation of the Achilles tendon, which is stretched beyond its capacity, or overused to the point where it begins to wear down and weaken, thereby becoming inflamed and/or torn away from either the back part of the heel bone to which it is attached, or the place where it becomes the lower end of the two calf muscles—the *gastrocnemius* and the *soleus* (see Diagram 8:6). In some cases the fault is not that of an Achilles tendon that is overstressed or too short, but of a shortened calf muscle that forces the tendon to overstretch to make up for the imbalance.

DIAGRAM 8:6
The Achilles Tendon

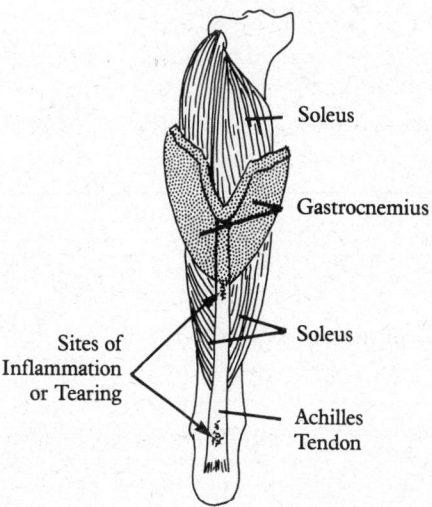

Soleus

Gastrocnemius

Soleus

Sites of
Inflammation
or Tearing

Achilles
Tendon

There are numerous ways of determining the cause of the tendonitis, and much of the diagnosis is based on taking the patient's medical history properly. Has the problem existed since childhood? Is there a history in adulthood of the condition? Has the problem begun since an athletic endeavor was undertaken? Has the patient recently switched from predominantly high-heeled shoes to low-heeled shoes? Has the patient suffered some sort of traumatic injury? Another important factor to be considered is that of abnormal pronation or abnormal supination. Are faulty biomechanics to blame for the disorder, either separately or in conjunction with another cause?

How can the ubiquitous biomechanical fault cause Achilles tendonitis? When the Achilles tendon *fires* (is activated) it pulls the foot into *plantar flexion* (that is, it lowers the front part of the foot towards the ground). When a person is running, or otherwise engaged in athletic activities, the calf muscles act to decelerate the lower leg and foot (that is, when the heel is planted on the ground, the calf muscles prevent the lower leg from going forward too fast and causing an imbalance). This action of the calf muscles strains the Achilles tendon—but not abnormally, unless a problem exists. That problem could be either abnormal pronation or abnormal supination of the foot, which tilts the heel bone to the inside or the outside. When that happens, the Achilles tendon will be pulled, perhaps beyond its comfortable limit, to compensate for the tilting heel bone. I see this syndrome often at the Sports Medicine Clinic at Toronto's Mount Sinai Hospital, particularly in runners and tennis players—for reasons I shall discuss fully in the chapters dealing with sports medicine.

Pain in the Achilles tendon will vary in location depending on where the inflammation and/or tearing is occurring. If the tendon is being overstressed where it joins with the two calf muscles, the discomfort will be felt in the lower leg; if the problem exists where the tendon attaches to the heel bone, the pain will be felt in that area. The worst possible thing that can happen to the Achilles tendon is a rupture, either complete or partial. When the tendon is torn in half, for whatever reason, the sensation is one of being shot in the back of the leg—according to many victims, who also report that they heard a loud pop when it happened. The pain is accompanied by a feeling of paralysis in the lower leg and foot, since the severed tendon provides no essential locomotion for the lower limb.

Becoming Well-Heeled: Part II

As I mentioned earlier in this chapter, treatment of an Achilles tendon is not easy, primarily because poor blood supply to the area prevents essential nutrients from reaching the soft tissues in sufficient amounts to promote healing. So, how does one get rid of the inflammation?

The first course of action, after the proper diagnosis and cause of the disorder has been established, is physiotherapy.

Ultrasound is the first choice at present. The sound waves convert to heat waves once they are deep into the soft tissues of the body, and they promote the opening of the blood vessels in the area to allow more blood and nutrients to reach the inflammation and work to heal it. Ultrasound used for this purpose tends to work better if it is applied after the area has been heated up and stretched for a few minutes. The heat will open up the blood vessels even more, and thus allow more blood into the area to aid in the healing process. This routine serves to open the vessels wider than if the ultrasound were used alone.

A method of treatment currently gaining favor is the use of *friction rubs*, particularly in the case of a chronic condition. Friction rubs work like some forms of massage, particularly *Shiatsu*, and, in fact, inflame the sore area even more. The idea is to trick the body into attacking the inflammation with added vigor. If that happens, the inflammation will theoretically heal faster on its own, without the need for other forms of treatment. I believe that this is another positive example of making nature do work that is often left to medication and direct intervention.

Once therapy, whatever the form, has succeeded in calming the inflammation, stretching exercises can begin to lengthen both the Achilles tendon and the calf muscles, if that is necessary. However, it would be wise to warm up the muscles and the tendon first, for two reasons. First, cold soft-tissue can itself be damaged if stretched too far; secondly, warm soft-tissue can be stretched to its maximum, thereby allowing for optimum results in the stretching program. Your therapist will show you how to do these exercises properly.

Again, one method of treatment I avoid is the use of anti-inflammatory drugs, either the injection of cortisone into the inflamed area, or the taking of non-steroidal pills. First, cortisone injected into the area of the Achilles tendon may get rid of the inflammation, but it may also cause the tendon to rupture by fraying it badly. We at the Sports Medicine Clinic have never injected cortisone into the tendon since we opened the clinic. Secondly, because of the poor circulation to the area, I feel that the use of anti-inflammatory drugs taken orally is a waste of time. In order for the drug to reach the inflammation in a dosage large enough to have an effect, it would have to be taken in almost toxic amounts. The cure would be far worse than the disease.

In extreme cases—most likely those of athletes who refuse to rest when afflicted by Achilles tendonitis—where the usual conservative treatments have not worked, it may be necessary to totally immobilize the tendon by placing the lower leg and foot in a plaster cast. This prevents a person from moving the tendon at all, and allows the Achilles tendon the opportunity to heal. The cast may have to be left on for six to twelve weeks, depending on the severity of the damage, and a lengthy physiotherapy program will be required after it has been removed so that the tendon and the surrounding muscles can regain their normal strength and flexibility.

The only other time the area may have to be placed in a cast is if the Achilles tendon has been ruptured. If the tendon is severed, it will have to be sewn together, because poor blood circulation to the area will hinder natural healing. Once the surgery has been completed, the leg will be placed in a "below-knee" cast to prevent any motion of the tendon for about six to eight weeks, while the area heals. As you can imagine, a lengthy physiotherapy program will follow.

Let us assume, however, that the damage is not that severe, and that the inflammation has been controlled by physiotherapy and rest. What happens when it is determined that the primary cause of the inflammation is biomechanical? Well, you have probably guessed that an orthotic device should be prescribed and placed in the shoe as quickly as possible to prevent further inflammation. Orthotic devices are not total cures, because the tendon still must be stretched to normal length. However, the devices allow the tendon to pull at a proper angle relative to the heel bone and the calf muscles. This is because the device will correct the abnormal pronation or abnormal supination that has been causing the inflammation.

At our Sports Medicine Clinic we have treated close to a hundred and fifty cases of Achilles tendonitis with orthotic devices, in conjunction with physiotherapy, when the patient has had a history of at least one year of the condition without receiving relief from other treatments. Our success rate has been about eighty-five per cent.

The Cinderella Syndrome

You are obviously aware of the story of Cinderella, the poor waif whose life changed dramatically when a piece of footwear transformed her miserable life into one of love and luxury. What the fairy tale did not tell you is that she had a great deal of anguish whenever she wore her glass slipper because it irritated the back of her foot terribly. She may well have been the first known celebrity to have suffered from *pump bump* (in medicalese, *Haglund's deformity*), which is a condition caused by irritation to the Achilles-tendon area of the foot. The primary suspect is the "pump"—the two-to-four-inch high-heeled shoe that is low-cut and has no straps or ties. While these shoes may be fashionable, they are hardly practical when foot comfort is involved.

The back of the offending shoe is usually slightly curved to cut directly into the back part of the heel bone, which may already be under some stress from an abnormally short Achilles tendon pulling on it. As with the case of plantar fasciitis, in which the front part of the heel will develop a ridge, or spurs, to shorten the distance between it and the metatarsal heads, a similar *exostosis* (protuberance of bony or cartilage-like material) may form at the back of the heel to compensate for the stress on a short Achilles tendon. This benign growth is called a "pump bump", and because of the constant irritation of the area around the bump, an inflammation can develop. This irritation is normally the result of "pump" shoes, or in a few cases of ski boots or skates. In any event, about ninety-five per cent of the cases of pump bump that I see are women.

The inflammation caused by a pump bump can occasionally occur not only to the heel bone itself, and/or to the Achilles tendon, but to the *bursa* (see Diagram 8:7). A bursa is a small sack of fibrous tissue that is filled with fluid and acts to protect parts of the body that are being irritated by friction, or by some other abnormal internal or external pressure, usually that which occurs between tendon or other soft tissue and bone (for example, in joints). However, bursae can themselves become inflamed, and the result is *bursitis*, a condition that can produce sharp pain and tenderness in the afflicted area.

DIAGRAM 8:7
The Pump Bump and Bursa Locations

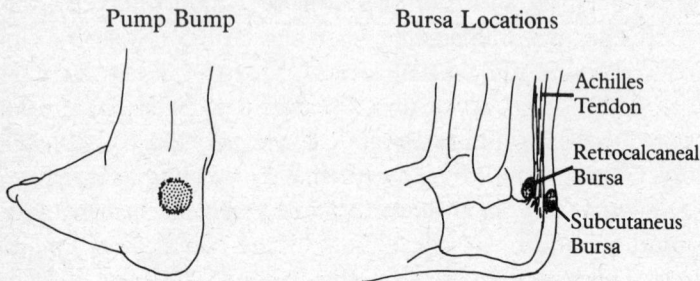

Pump Bump   Bursa Locations

Achilles
Tendon

Retrocalcaneal
Bursa

Subcutaneus
Bursa

There are two types of bursitis that can occasionally affect the area around a pump bump: *retro-calcaneal* and *subcutaneus*. The former occurs between tendon and bone, the second between tendon and skin (also Diagram 8:7). These conditions are not easy to distinguish from Achilles tendonitis, and the feel and knowledge of an experienced foot specialist is often required to make the proper diagnosis.

Bursitis in this part of the body can be treated by ice, ultrasound, and the wearing of proper footwear, since the condition is exacerbated, if not directly caused, by shoe pressure which pushes tendon against bone, or against other soft tissue. Since I see only three or four cases a year, I would not worry too much about falling victim to this benign disorder. As I mentioned above, the major problem with bursitis in the back of the foot is diagnosis, not treatment.

When the problem is with the pump bump itself, and not the bursa, the treatment is generally much the same—ice, ultrasound, and a change of footwear. However, another possibility is the use of a *donut pad* that can be applied directly to the sore area at the back of the foot, or to the shoe, ski boot, or skate. This will alleviate the pressure being applied directly to the inflammation. I know many athletes who wear these pads regularly to protect themselves from a pump bump. The use of an orthotic device may also be indicated if the condition involves an Achilles tendon that is too short and affects the biomechanics of the lower leg and foot.

In very rare cases—about two per cent of the time—surgery will be required to rid the patient of the inflammation. Usually the offending bump of bone is removed by being filed down. The procedure can be done under a local anesthetic in a doctor's office using either an open or an M.I.S. technique. Recovery is normally quite rapid and uncomplicated.

In the rarer cases, in which the Achilles tendon is actually attached to the heel bone where the pump bump has developed, the tendon will have to be removed surgically from the bone, and then reattached after the bump has been filed down. As you can imagine, this is a more complicated procedure, and the foot will have to be placed in a cast for six to twelve weeks to facilitate healing. Before you begin to worry about this happening to you, be comforted in the fact that this type of surgery is required in less than one per cent of all incidents of pump bump.

The Dark at the Middle of the Tunnel
I want to talk now about a nerve-impingement condition called the *tarsal-tunnel syndrome*. The tunnel in question runs down the back part of the lower leg into the foot, and is a small, bony passageway for the *tibialis posterior nerve* that bifurcates (branches out) into two separate nerves in the foot—the *medial plantar nerve* and the *lateral plantar nerve*. You may recall this nerve system from the chapter on the anatomy of the foot and lower leg.

As you can see from Diagram 8:8, the tarsal tunnel runs under the *deltoid ligament*. When something is amiss with the ligament, and it is forced to impinge on the tarsal tunnel, or if the tunnel is otherwise constricted, the tibialis posterior nerve is squeezed and *entrapped*. The agitated nerve then begins to send out confusing signals to the brain—numbness, a feeling of pins and needles, burning sensations on the bottom of the foot, and/or a stabbing pain in the area of the ankle. Because of these vague, diffused symptoms, the tarsal-tunnel syndrome is difficult to diagnose, particularly since the symptoms are often non-existent when the deltoid ligament is at rest (that is, when the person is not exercising or walking). The resting ligament will not impinge on the nerve as it passes through the tarsal tunnel.

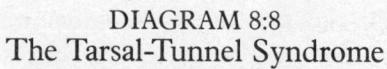

DIAGRAM 8:8
The Tarsal-Tunnel Syndrome

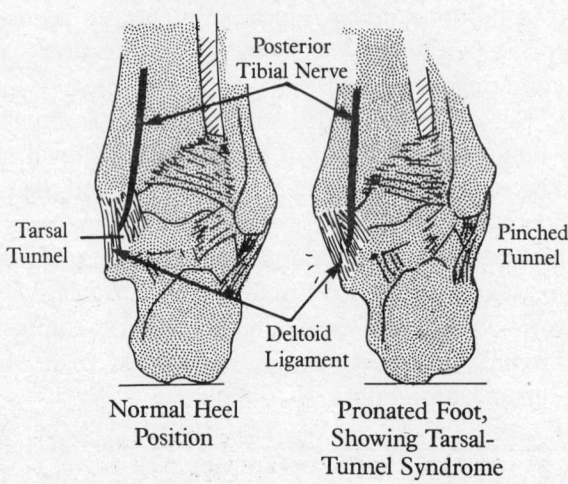

Posterior
Tibial Nerve

Tarsal
Tunnel

Pinched
Tunnel

Deltoid
Ligament

Normal Heel
Position

Pronated Foot,
Showing Tarsal-
Tunnel Syndrome

The primary cause of the tarsal-tunnel syndrome is our old enemy, the biomechanical fault. When a foot is severely over-pronating, the deltoid ligament is forced to assume an abnormal position to compensate. When it is forced into the position shown at the right in Diagram 8:8, the ligament pushes down on the tarsal tunnel, thereby indirectly impinging on the tibialis posterior nerve—and causing the tarsal-tunnel syndrome.

The second major cause of the disorder is systemic—actually a whole host of systemic disorders—serious or mild, temporary or permanent. When an ankle swells, because of water retention, poor circulation, or even pregnancy (when poor circulation in the pelvic area can result in similar difficulties in the lower limbs), entrapment of the nerve can occur, caused by the fact that the space allowed for the tarsal tunnel has been restricted. Only about twenty-five per cent of the cases I see in my practice are systemically induced. I would suspect that the percentages of the two causes would be dramatically reversed in an obstetrician's practice. Since I see only six or seven cases of the syndrome in a year, it is not likely that I would ever have an office full of pregnant women with a nerve-impingement problem in their lower legs.

As I have already mentioned, diagnosing the syndrome is a real pain—for the doctor. When the patient is resting, there is a good chance the problem will not be evident at all, since the deltoid ligament causing the discomfort is relaxed, and therefore not stressing the tarsal tunnel. I often ask my active patients who experience the discomfort only when running or engaged in other exercise to go out and run or exercise and then return to my office once the pain begins—if they can make it back. I advise them to take taxi fare with them in case they manage to produce excruciating pain while trying to induce the symptoms. When the patients have returned in agony to my office, I am then more able to seek out the cause of the problem by conducting various nerve-entrapment tests that are themselves painless.

If I find that the problem is tarsal-tunnel syndrome, and if the problem is obviously systemic, and accompanied by swollen ankles, I send the patients on to be seen by other specialists for further diagnosis and treatment. If, on the other hand, I establish that the cause is biomechanical, I can begin treating the patient.

As you would suspect, the proper treatment for biomechanically induced tarsal-tunnel syndrome is correction of the biomechanical fault. If the condition is relatively mild, a simple arch-support and/or switching to a well-constructed running-shoe (for the patient who does not constantly require formal footwear) should do the trick. If the disorder is more severe, a special orthotic device will have to be fitted. Anti-inflammatory drugs to control the discomfort are of little use, because of poor blood circulation to the area of the discomfort. Physiotherapy, such as the application of ice or ultrasound, may help if the ankle itself has become swollen after having been injured in some way.

9

Itchy Feet: Dermatological Foot Problems

Starting from Scratch

The study of skin diseases—*dermatology*—is a very difficult science. One of the problems in identifying a condition is picking the correct option from the thousands that exist. A full catalogue of skin diseases would fill a medical textbook. Also, the disorders come in a multitude of varieties, and erupt on just about any part of the body. Another problem is that of research. Skin diseases are rarely fatal; therefore, there is rarely a pressing need to find a miracle cure for a condition that may well eventually go away by itself or respond by some chance to medications or other treatments that already exist.

So there is one general rule of thumb for the treatment of skin disorders, and I learned it from one of my medical-school professors of dermatology: if it's wet, dry it; if it's dry, wet it.

Fortunately, most skin disorders of the foot are quite easy to identify, and can generally be dealt with successfully by using the present state-of-the-art in treatments. However, I am occasionally puzzled by a condition that defies logic. For example, I have one female patient who constantly complains of a tiny itchy spot on the side of one foot, in the area of the heel bone. The skin is not inflamed and there are no other symptoms of any systemic disorder. I suspect the problem is an allergic reaction, since the itch is not always present, but I have no idea what that allergy may be. However, since the patient's only major problem to date has been to scratch holes in her pantyhose, neither of us wishes to investigate the condition further.

I have already discussed in previous chapters certain conditions that might be considered dermatological. These would include corns, calluses, and warts. I would readily agree that plantar warts are dermatological disorders, but I decided arbitrarily to include them in the chapter dealing with conditions affecting the bottom of the foot. Corns and calluses are caused by biomechanical faults and, as such, ought to be discussed apart from other skin problems of the foot. So, what does that leave for this chapter? Well, as you might imagine, there is at least one major skin disorder that almost exclusively attacks the foot, and that is *tinea pedis*. Translated literally from the Latin, tinea pedis means "a fungus of the foot", not "a tin foot". We know it most commonly as *athlete's foot*.

The Case of the Mushrooming Foreign Agent: Athlete's Foot
I could never quite figure out how tinea pedis became known as athlete's foot, although I suspect it had something to do with the fact that the foreign agent responsible for all the trouble lurks in hot, dark, moist places like an athlete's changing-room locker. The disease affects athletes and non-athletes alike, and plays no favorites. I have seen cases of athlete's foot in infants as young as six months, and in people as old as ninety-five.

A fungus is a very opportunistic agent; a damp towel, a sweaty shoe or sock, or other moist clothing, can keep it going and growing for days, often until it can transfer to a part of the human body. Two of these fungi, the *trichophyton mentagrophyte* and the *trichophyton rubrum*, seek a home in the skin of the foot. These fungi can flourish on the foot because the conditions are perfect for their growth—moist, dark, and hot. Once the fungi establish a foothold, they can be tough to dislodge, particularly if the victim waits a long time before seeking relief.

Athlete's foot can happen to the healthiest of feet, but it is not contagious unless the proper conditions exist. The fungus can hide in a wet piece of clothing or towel until it comes in contact with a foot that readily accepts it and promotes its growth by providing a dark, sweaty, safe haven. For some unknown reason, certain people seem to have a built-in immunity to fungal infections, while others need only look at a mildewy towel to wind up with athlete's foot. At the health club to which I belong, I see many men walking around the changing area, the showers, and the pools wearing shower sandals in order to protect their feet from the fungus. And they still succumb to the disease. Others walk blithely barefoot throughout the entire area and never have the slightest hint of a fungal infection. Unfortunately, if you are one of the sufferers, there appears to be a connection between athlete's foot and fungal nails, and they may constantly reinfect each other.

I have had a few patients ask me if athlete's foot can spread throughout the body. The family of fungi to which the mentagrophytes belong can make themselves at home anywhere on the body where the proper conditions exist for them to mushroom. However, since the leg itself is neither hot, moist, nor dark compared to the foot or, for example, the groin, it would be unlikely that the fungal infection would spread all the way from a victim's foot up the leg. It would be rare to find a fungal infection that did not confine itself to the more hospitable parts of the foot, although I do occasionally see a common fungal infection of the foot and groin, and, less often, a trychophyton rubrum infection of hair follicles on the legs.

The athlete's-foot infection is found sixty per cent of the time between the third and fourth toes, or the fourth and fifth toes. I have a theory why this is so, and it involves the so-called soft, or wet, corn that can develop in those areas because of the friction caused by one toe rubbing against the other. It is not always easy for non-experts to differentiate between a wet corn and a fungal infection, and in the majority of cases they choose the corn. So the unsuspecting sufferer will often apply medicated corn pads to the area. But these home remedies contain acids that can burn the skin and destroy its natural defences against a fungal infection. Not only is the area moist, dark, and hot, it is also weakened by the acid and is therefore much more susceptible to a fungal infection. The poor victim may then wind up with two problems, if indeed a wet corn did exist: the corn and the fungal infection. I see about ten such cases a year, almost all with the two disorders between the fourth and fifth toes.

Although athlete's foot will normally develop first between toes, it can initially break out on the sole of the foot, particularly under the metatarsal heads on the ball of the foot. Of course, it may well spread rapidly from between the toes to the bottom of the foot, or vice versa.

The infected area itself is well defined by a reddish line around it. Inside the line is a whitish flaking of skin where the fungus is growing. It has the appearance of onion-skin peeling, and the discomfort it causes is enough to make you cry. This peeling is nature's way of trying to rid itself of the fungus, but it does not work, because the foreign agent is too tenacious. Anyone who has suffered from athlete's foot can attest to the fact that the condition produces severe itching. Many sufferers complain of a nasty burning sensation, particularly when the fungus invades the bottom of the foot. Put all these symptoms together and it becomes easier to differentiate between wet corns and athlete's foot.

The two trychophytons that commonly cause athlete's foot may also appear in different areas with different symptoms. The rubrum fungus usually infects the toe-web (between the toes), and causes a dry scaling. The mentagrophyte fungus usually appears on the instep in the form of *vesicles* (small blisters), and tends to be a more inflammatory type of athlete's foot.

Slow and Steady Does Not Win the Day

The trick to defeating the athlete's-foot fungus is to catch it early. Fortunately, an attack on the fungus does not require expensive medicines and lengthy waits in a doctor's office. Now that you know what causes the problem, and how you can identify it, a little common sense and the application of over-the-counter anti-fungal agents can solve it before it becomes a major dilemma.

There is a billion-dollar business going on that has mushroomed out of the need for non-prescriptive, over-the-counter, anti-fungal medication. Fortunately, most of these preparations do work quite well when you also eliminate the conditions that the fungi thrive on. They come in a variety of sprays, creams, powders, and soaks, and are most effective when applied immediately after the onset of the fungal infection. The area affected by the fungus must also be kept cool and in the light whenever possible. Those three conditions may not always be easy to attain, particularly if you have to be outdoors during the winter months. In warm weather, someone with athlete's foot ought to be able to remain sockless and barefoot at least part of the day, although such footwear—or lack of it—could cause problems at the office.

Aside from taking all the above steps to defeat the fungus, you should also soak a foot with a fungal infection in a solution of salt and warm water. The saline solution helps provide an unappealing atmosphere for the fungus and softens the affected skin, thereby enabling the anti-fungal preparations applied after the saline bath to penetrate deeper and act more effectively. Also, the salt and water will dry the skin somewhat, so that excess perspiration can be prevented.

My wine-loving friend also has a foot balm for treating athlete's foot. His potion consists of an ounce of sage, an ounce of agrimony (a herbal plant), and two cups of white wine. The concoction is heated, but not boiled, for twenty minutes while covered. The affected foot is then soaked in it repeatedly. Here he becomes vague about timing, but I assume that when the foot hiccups, it has been soaked long enough.

Because the athlete's-foot fungus can live for up to fourteen days on the insole of some shoes, it would be wise, as a preventive measure, to spray the shoes with an anti-fungal preparation, particularly if you have a history of fungal infections.

If you take all the above steps, you have a seventy-five-per-cent chance of success in treating athlete's foot, as long as you have not allowed the infection to progress for days. But if the condition has become acute, or has been allowed to linger for too long, stronger medications will be required, and they must be dispensed by prescription. There are six or seven of these stronger preparations available in North America, and they are generally quite effective— once again as long as all the other measures mentioned above are taken. Should all topical medications prove unsuccessful, it may be necessary to turn to the pill as a last resort. The pill in this case is an anti-fungal drug, and it is highly successful in treating athlete's foot. Unfortunately, these pills can also play havoc with your system, and for that reason I am most reluctant to prescribe them.

Partners in Crime

Misery loves company, and the discomfort of athlete's foot can be made worse by the simultaneous infection of the area by bacterial agents that love to attack already-weakened sites on the body. Once the fungus has breached the skin, the way is open for all types of alien agents. When a bacterial and a fungal infection flourish in the same place at the same time, it will be necessary to use a double-barrelled approach to kill them both. Some of the over-the-counter preparations are both anti-fungal and anti-bacterial, and they work quite well. Of course, other steps must also be taken to keep the area dry, cool, and light. If you treat one condition but not the other, a ping-pong situation will develop. First, the one healthy infection will pave the way for the return of the other, and the game will seesaw back and forth until both are attacked simultaneously.

Occasionally a third villain enters the fray. When a part of the foot has been attacked by fungi and bacteria over a reasonable amount of time, the affected area will also become inflamed. If that happens, you must then add a third barrel to the shotgun: a steroid topical preparation (a cortisone-type cream) to handle the inflammation. Quite a few drug companies have now combined the three medicines into one topical cream, and many of them seem to work well. They are all prescription drugs.

It is important to tackle the inflammation quickly, because the more inflamed the skin, the more hospitable it is to fungal and bacterial infections. Many dermatologists and podiatrists are fairly skeptical about these new three-way creams; I will prescribe them only when all the other treatments have failed. The reason for the skepticism is that medical professionals believe that anti-inflammatory steroid medications aid the development of a bacterial or fungal infection in these cases. There is also a high incidence of allergy to the preservatives and/or the neomycin found in these creams.

Return of the Fungi
Most of the patients I see with athlete's foot naturally want to know if the disease will return once it has been cured. The answer is affirmative. If the same conditions exist that allowed the fungus to attack the foot in the first place, it will strike again, but more often in some people than in others. I mentioned above that there are those who are more prone to athlete's foot than others. The problem may be one of life-style—too much time spent in health-club locker rooms—but I suspect that it is one of body chemistry. Just as certain people attract mosquitoes and blackflies, while others do not, certain people seem to send out welcome signals to fungi.

If you seem susceptible to fungal infections in general, it would be wise to follow some of the preventive measures I outlined when talking about the treatment of athlete's foot. Be careful when you are in public showering and locker-room areas. Take extra care to keep your feet dry and cool, and spray your footwear regularly with anti-fungal preparations. Try to avoid footwear that has been treated to keep water out, for it also prevents the foot from "breathing", thereby trapping perspiration and creating a warm, moist spot for a fungus to grow. The same applies to one of the latest crazes in women's footwear, plastic shoes. These shoes appear to be responsible for a recent minor increase in fungal infections in women's feet.

One final bit of advice: If you have identified the problem as athlete's foot, but the over-the-counter preparations fail to provide relief, get to a doctor before the infection spreads and picks up partners in crime.

Contact Dermatitis

One of the often baffling mysteries in medicine is what causes *contact dermatitis*, an inflammation of the skin. The inflammation is caused by a foreign agent, but it is neither a fungus nor a bacterium. It is a type of chemical or a combination of things to which you may be allergic. Often the culprit is easy to identify, but at other times it may take days of investigation to pick it out over other suspects. One easy identification would probably include an article of clothing or footwear made of fibers to which you may be allergic. As an example, there are many people who cannot tolerate black dye (paraphenylene diamine) next to their skin. Take away the black dye and the contact dermatitis disappears almost immediately.

But often the problem lies with a chemical, or a combination of chemicals, that may be found in soaps, detergents, perfumes, dyes, glues, or tanning agents that have been used in making a pair of shoes. At other times a systemic allergic reaction to a drug or a food may make the skin ultra-sensitive to things that would not normally irritate it. To compound the puzzle, there are so many new synthetics and combinations of synthetics on the market today in clothing, footwear, cleaning products, and food that the search for the allergen becomes similar to a search for a needle in a haystack. So, when a medical professional is dealing with contact dermatitis, you can see why he or she often has to play the role of detective.

It is often quite easy to pinpoint the general cause of contact dermatitis of the foot. If the outbreak occurs specifically when you wear a new pair of shoes or stockings, they will become the primary suspects. However, it is usually far from easy to clearly identify what it is in the footwear that is producing the dermatitis. And even when the investigator is lucky enough to identify the chemical involved, how can you, the patient, avoid it in the future when you buy new shoes and stockings? How many shoe or stocking sales-personnel know precisely the composition of each item they have in their store? Fortunately, shoe manufacturers have been co-operating with dermatologists and podiatrists in revealing all the materials that have gone into the making of their products. But the list of materials is large, and not all people react adversely to the same chemicals or combinations thereof.

While shoes and stockings are the primary culprits in the outbreak of contact dermatitis, there are other foreign agents that can cause similar problems, and I have already mentioned most of them—detergents, soaps, and perfumes being the most common. I had one case recently that had me baffled for quite a while until the patient told me about her Mother's Day present.

This women had a terrible case of contact dermatitis all over both feet, even though she had not recently purchased any new footwear or a new type of stocking. For a while she consented to wear only wooden shoes with no stockings, but the dermatitis remained and, in fact, worsened.

Both her dermatologist and I examined her and were puzzled. We could not find any systemic cause for her rash, and she told us repeatedly that she had not changed laundry detergents or bath soap. But one day she admitted that, as a Mother's Day gift, she had received a popular foot cream that is applied after a bath, and she had been using it daily ever since. The onset of the dermatitis coincided with the use of the cream. The moment she stopped using the cream, the rash began to clear up by itself. There was obviously a chemical in the preparation to which she was acutely allergic. Sometimes it pays to look a gift-horse in the mouth.

It is easier to identify contact dermatitis on the foot than it is to find the causative agent. It can occur almost anywhere on the foot and is usually a flat rash with red pinpoints. It will erupt fairly quickly after exposure to the irritant or allergen, usually within twenty-four to thirty-six hours, but occasionally sooner if the allergy is a strong one. It is often seen precisely where a strap of a shoe, like a sandal, cuts across the bare part of the foot. The area not directly in contact with the shoe will be perfectly normal. The reaction could be compared to that of a tornado that wreaks havoc over a precisely defined area while leaving adjacent strips of land unscathed.

Once the condition has been diagnosed and the cause discovered, the treatment of contact dermatitis is fairly routine. First, you remove the irritant and try to avoid it in the future. Cortisone-type creams applied to the affected area will help relieve the inflammation. In Canada these creams must be prescribed by a doctor. Also, it helps to soak the affected foot in salt and warm water. The soaking opens the pores and allows the cortisone preparation to penetrate deeper under the surface, thereby enhancing its healing capabilities. Also, the soaking helps prevent the development of a secondary bacterial infection.

There are many other types of dermatitis that can affect the foot, some of them caused by systemic disorders and others by contact with something to which the person may be allergic. However, contact dermatitis is the most common of the lot, and it would serve no useful purpose in this book to try and list all the others, along with their diagnoses, causes, and treatments. My advice to anyone who has a dermatological problem on the foot is to seek the opinion of a specialist, either a podiatrist or a dermatologist, if the condition does not begin to clear up within a couple of days.

Not Just a Friendly, Furry Animal
We turn now to the subject of *moles*, and straight away I want to assure you that they are rarely malignant. So you need not cower with fright as you read the following few paragraphs.

A mole is a small, permanent area of *pigmentation* (discoloration) on the skin. It is usually brownish in color. Some moles are flat, some are raised; some have hairs growing out of them, others do not. Why they develop in the first place is a moot point; why they change in rare cases from benign to malignant has kept researchers busy for years.

Moles can appear anywhere on the foot. But when they exist on the bottom of the foot, or between the toes, they may be more susceptible to irritation, and many experts feel that when a mole is being constantly irritated it is more likely to present problems than if it sits peacefully unbothered. In any event, only one mole out of a hundred thousand will ever turn into a *malignant melanoma*.

Unfortunately, we are being told by researchers that melanomas are the second-fastest-growing form of cancer after lung cancer. This is thought to be related to overexposure to the sun. There is a mistaken belief in many communities that a tanned body is a healthier one.

When it comes to moles on the feet, I believe that if the possibility of constant irritation exists, they ought to be removed for safety's sake. They can be excised easily in a doctor's office under a local anesthetic, and the site will require only a couple of stitches to close. It is a tiny price to pay for a sound preventive measure.

In general, I believe that all new moles ought to be examined by a doctor. The same applies to any existing mole that suddenly begins growing, changing color, or bleeding, or that becomes sensitive. It is most important to remember, however, that the odds are strongly in your favor that any mole you may have will never cause you any trouble.

The Heartbreak of Psoriasis
I can recall seeing advertisements on television a few years ago for a preparation used to treat *psoriasis*, and it sympathetically referred to the disease as heartbreaking, probably because it can be quite disfiguring to the skin when it is severe. Psoriasis is a skin disease that can apparently be hereditary and is the result of an abnormal over-production of *keratin* by the body. Keratin is a fibrous protein that is essential in the development of healthy skin and nails. As you will discover in the next chapter, psoriasis can affect either skin or nails, or both at the same time. Although we hear a lot about psoriasis, it affects no more than two per cent of the North American population. Unfortunately, those who do suffer from the disease often have a miserable time because it is very difficult to treat and it has a nasty habit of recurring.

Psoriasis is characterized by itchy, scaly, red patches, and occurs most often on parts of the body where there are bony protuberances, such as on the elbow or on the knee. As far as the foot is concerned, psoriasis is most likely to be found where a bony area is being constantly irritated. Common sites are on pump bumps, bunions, and the soles of the feet.

The disease is not confined to people who are "unwell"; it can strike even the healthiest person. One of the reasons may be that stress might be a contributing factor, or even environmental problems. However, there is still much research to be done in these areas before the environment can be blamed for either causing or aggravating psoriatic outbreaks. (I will, though, ask a patient with psoriasis if he or she has undergone some type of emotional stress during the time in which the condition appeared.) As well as stress, a systemic infection caused by *strep* bacteria can also occasionally trigger an episode of psoriasis.

There are two interesting features that help in the diagnosis of psoriasis—and the diagnosis is not always easy because the disease can mimic other dermatological disorders, such as dermatitis. One feature is called *Koebner's phenomenon.* If the psoriatic area is traumatized or burned, the lesion will return along with the new growth of skin. This is not the case with most other skin disorders. The second unique aspect of psoriasis is that when the overlying thick, silvery, scaly material is removed from the affected area, there will be pinpoint bleeding underneath it. This is known in medicalese as *Auspitz's sign.*

There is more than one type of psoriasis, unfortunately, and that makes diagnosis of the disease even more complicated. As far as the foot is concerned, one of the most common forms is known as *pustular psoriasis.* It affects the soles of the feet (and the palms of the hands) and appears without a trace of any other form of the disease in the area. The affected part of the skin will be covered by a scaly patch, beneath which are tiny *pustules,* or water-filled white, gray, or yellow blisters. The disorder can be confused with various infections, so it is necessary to take a culture of the lesions. If the culture proves to be negative for any type of infection, a diagnosis of pustular psoriasis can be made with a fair degree of accuracy.

A complication of psoriasis is *psoriatic arthritis,* which is definitely a systemic disease rather than a wear-and-tear process. However, only a very small percentage of patients with psoriasis ever contract it. The disease may manifest itself as a mild outbreak on the finger joints, or it can be severe and generalized throughout the body, mimicking rheumatoid arthritis. Because of its nature, I believe that psoriatic arthritis ought to be placed in the hands of a rheumatologist for proper evaluation and treatment.

Breaking the Heart of Psoriasis

Psoriasis is not an easy disorder to treat right now, although I believe that researchers will catch up to the disease in the next few years. But until the time when the exact causes of the disease are isolated, we shall have to rely on controlling the symptoms. At present, there is no known cure for psoriasis.

One of the most effective treatments seems to be exposing the affected area to sunlight. This may be difficult in mid-winter in northern climes, but in the warm months of the year a person with psoriasis on the feet ought to try to get as much sun on the affected area as possible. However, be careful not to wind up with a sunburn in the process. If sunlight is not readily available or you prefer not to expose yourself to it, one alternative is ultraviolet-ray therapy. This type of light seems to have a similar effect to sunlight when it comes to controlling psoriasis. But this treatment is not a cure either.

There are some topical preparations that will also provide relief. The cortisone family of skin creams will often help, as will the application of coal-tar preparations, or anthralin.

If none of the above works, there are alternatives that dermatologists can prescribe, such as methotrexate, retinoids, or psoralens with ultraviolet light (U.V.A.) (better known as P.U.V.A. therapy). What I try to tell my patients with stubborn cases of psoriasis is to try and keep the disease under control with non-systemic treatments, and to be patient. My dermatologist colleagues assure me that more effective treatments are close at hand.

Sweating It Out

Like the rest of the body, there are sweat glands under the skin of the feet. Also, there is a normal assortment of bacteria on the skin of the feet. When perspiration combines with certain types of bacteria, the result is a bad odor. This odor can be enhanced by environmental conditions, such as hot, humid weather, and the breathability of shoes and stockings. Some people are not bothered by malodorous feet—their own or those of others. But many are disturbed by their own offensive body odors, and those of people with whom they come in contact. Judging by the number of patients I have who complain about their own foot odors, the latter group are in the majority, if my patients can be considered a cross-section of North American society.

Sweat glands right under the skin secrete the body's nitrogenous wastes. Perspiration is also nature's way of keeping the body's temperature from becoming too high. Thus, when a person has a fever, he or she perspires in an attempt to lower body temperature to normal. This form of perspiration also combines with certain bacteria usually found on the skin to produce an unpleasant odor.

In a sense, then, we are left with a dilemma. How can we allow nature to do what comes naturally, but at the same time prevent unpleasant body odors? I will almost always come down on the side of allowing the body to function normally. However, this does not mean that nothing can be done to prevent body odor.

Sweat glands are particularly abundant in the armpits—hence the multi-billion-dollar business of underarm anti-perspirants and deodorants—and on the soles of the feet. This is why our feet appear to perspire more than most other parts of our body. While there is a variety of products on the market to control underarm odor, such is not the case for feet.

There are two primary ways of controlling foot odor. One way is to reduce perspiration with the application of an anti-perspirant that can be either sprayed on, rolled on, or rubbed into the skin. The products, most of which have aluminum chlorhydrate as their main ingredient, clog the skin pores and prevent sweat from reaching the surface of the skin. Most of them are also perfumed. While the reduction of perspiration on the sole of the foot may discourage bacteria from proliferating there, an anti-perspirant does not affect bacteria already thriving on the surface of the skin. Moreover, many people are allergic to the ingredients of most anti-perspirant products and may develop nasty rashes where the products have been applied. Most importantly, though, nature is being tampered with. Anti-perspirants prevent the natural cooling of the body and natural elimination of waste products. Therefore, I would seek other means of coping with any foot-odor problem you may have.

Another approach is to try and change the type of bacteria flourishing on the foot. Some forms of bacteria are far more capable than others of producing unpleasant odors.

One method I recommend to my patients is to soak their feet three or four times daily in a saline solution. The solution will destroy certain types of bacteria that cause bad odors. After three or four weeks you may have far less of the odor-producing bacteria on the soles of your feet, and the situation may remain that way. An alternative to the saline solution is the application of rubbing alcohol. Follow the same instructions as with the saline solution, but allow the alcohol to dry on the surface of the skin.

Some people have the misfortune to perspire excessively on their feet. This condition is known as *hyperhydrosis*. Others may be plagued by excessively odiferous perspiration (*bromidrosis*). A combination of the two conditions is definitely unpleasant and not that easy to treat clinically.

If a person suffers from one or both of the above conditions, there is a surgical technique known as *sympathectomy*. This procedure involves cutting the nervous system that controls the sweat glands, and prevents the glands from reacting to nerve impulses that stimulate perspiration. I am totally opposed to this type of operation, because once again I believe that nature should not be tampered with in this way.

The logical approach to excessively sweaty, odiferous feet is to change shoes and socks as frequently as possible, as many as three or four times a day. This may sound impractical, but until a new, startling approach to the problem becomes available, you have little choice, short of what I consider to be uncalled-for surgery. You should be wearing socks made of natural fibers, such as cotton, because they are far more absorbent than synthetic materials. And you should wear shoes that allow the foot to breathe so that moisture has less chance of developing on your feet. There are some shoe inserts that claim to combat foot odor. If they help with your particular problem, there is nothing wrong with using them.

Some people have a very different disorder: they do not perspire enough. This condition is known as *anhidrosis*, and can either be congenital or be caused by some other existing disease.

A person with anhidrosis will suffer from very dry skin, because of a lack of necessary moisture on the bottom of the foot. This skin may become so dry as to crack or fissure, particularly in the heel area. The fissures may become infected if care is not taken to reduce the inflammation where the skin has cracked. Nails will also be affected by anhidrosis, and may actually begin to crack.

As I have mentioned earlier in the book, the best way to treat dry skin on the foot is to apply moisturizing creams twice daily to the affected areas. At night, before going to bed, a person can wrap the affected foot in a plastic wrap after the cream has been applied. This material is air-tight and will enhance absorption of the cream during the night because it acts to keep whatever perspiration there is on the skin. If there is an infection on the skin, or the risk of one, the application of an antibiotic cream is recommended along with the moisturizing cream. A pumice stone should be used on the affected areas after bathing or showering to remove dead skin-tissue from the foot. This will enhance the growth of new, healthier skin.

10
Right on the Nail

Nailing Down the Facts

A nail (*unguis*, in medicalese) is a horny covering that may have originally been nature's way of protecting the tip of a finger or a toe from injury or inflammation. It may also serve as an effective weapon, as any person who has ever been scratched by a sharp one can attest to. The forerunner of man might have used nails effectively to protect himself, or as a tool to provide food, shelter, and other essentials. This may be why the nail is one of the hardest parts of the human anatomy, and is so durable and potentially potent as a weapon. Of course, it is the fingernail that has proved so useful to mankind throughout the ages, but it is the toenail with which we are concerned in this chapter. So, enough about the use of the nail as a tool and a weapon. Keep in mind, though, that although there are differences between fingernails and toenails, they are also quite similar in many respects.

Nails are composed basically of *keratin*, a fibrous protein that grows out of the front part of the top of the toe and slides forward over the nail bed (see Diagram 10:1). As you can tell from the diagram, the whitish area at the bottom of the nail is called the *lunula* (a half-moon). The fold of skin lying directly above the *root* of the nail is the *nail fold*. (The root is also called the *nail matrix*, or *nail-growing plate*.) The layer of skin next to the nail root is called the *eponychium*. On your fingers you would recognize it as the cuticle.

The normal nail itself is clear; there ought to be no discoloration anywhere. And, as you can see in the diagram, a normal nail-growth

147

DIAGRAM 10:1
The Anatomy of a Nail

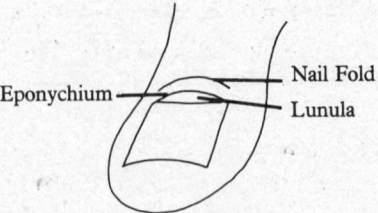

pattern should follow the actual contour of the toe. This is important to remember when cutting your nails.

Since the nail has no nerve endings, there is no pain directly associated with damage to the nail itself. If the nail is removed, either purposely or by accident, the discomfort felt is from the underlying tissue that has been traumatized. Once that tissue has healed, there will be no discomfort and the person who has lost the nail will be able to function quite normally. This is because the toenail really serves no useful function to modern man.

One major difference between the toenail and the fingernail is the growth period. Because blood-flow to the feet is not as good as it is to the hands, toenails grow to regular length at about one-third the pace of fingernails. Therefore, it takes about eighteen months for the development of a complete toenail.

There are numerous things that can go wrong with a toenail. Many of the problems produce discomfort, and may hinder normal walking. The people most commonly affected by nail disorders are those in the over-fifty age group, probably because they are more prone to accidental traumatization than most younger adults, and because they have had many years in which to develop and ignore conditions that can eventually cause problems.

As you will discover below, the most common cause of nail disorders is an insult, accidental or intentional, to a toe: stubbing it, dropping things on it, or having some heavy clod step on it. In most cases it is the big toe that is affected. That is because it just happens to be a bigger, better target than the others. Some nail disorders are caused by ill-fitting footwear, a faulty genetic make-up, or erratic nail-cutting. However, these are all exceptions rather than the norm.

By far the most common of all nail disorders is the ingrown toenail, so let us begin our discussion of what can go wrong with the nail by proceeding directly to this painful condition.

For Want of a Straight Nail
As you can see in Diagram 10:2, a normal toenail has no "incurvated" sides—that is, sides that grow into the toe itself rather than straight out. The *ingrown toenail (onychocryptosis)*, on the other hand, breaks the skin of the *nail wall* (also Diagram 10:2) and begins to grow into the toe itself. Contrary to popular belief—a belief unfortunately still held by too many medical professionals as well—ingrown toenails are not normally caused by improper cutting, or by wearing shoes that are too tight. Of course, one can definitely make the problem worse by wearing tight shoes, or by trying to cut fancy patterns in the toenail, but, as I have just mentioned, the major cause of ingrown toenails is trauma, somehow injuring the nail. Also, there are some people who have toenails that, for no particular reason, grow inward instead of straight out. Whatever the cause of the ingrown nail, quick attention is necessary to avoid lingering misery and the chance of acute infection. Such speedy action does not include bathroom surgery.

DIAGRAM 10:2
Cross-Section of a Normal and an Ingrown Nail

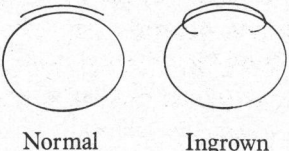

Normal   Ingrown

Ingrown toenails are not only the most common complaints of people with toenail problems, they also give rise to numerous old wives' tales about how they occur, and how they are best treated. We have already examined how they usually develop. But what exactly causes all the concern and discomfort? Well, one of the myths is that the nail itself hurts. As we pointed out at the beginning of the chapter, a nail has no nerve endings, so it cannot hurt.

The piece of nail that grows into the side of the nail bed and causes the discomfort is called a *spicule*. Once the spicule punctures and penetrates the skin, the area is open to bacterial growth. This is similar to having any foreign material, such as a sliver, penetrate the skin. The bacteria have a ready supply of fresh blood once they have found a hospitable home under the surface of the skin, and they can then produce a nice infection that will have to be treated with antibiotics.

The spicule penetrating the skin is made possible by the incurvated nail that has become curled for any one of a number of reasons. This incurvation becomes a chronic condition unless the proper treatment is used to permanently end the curling of the nail. Therefore, while it is helpful to treat the ingrown nail and its inherent infection with antibiotics and soaking, the root cause of the disorder will still have to be dealt with in order to prevent further infection and pain. I see patients on a regular basis who have been on almost continuous antibiotic therapy for ingrown toenail infections because they have not had the nail itself properly treated. Considering the potentially harmful effects and cost of regular antibiotic use, one could equate the therapy with that of brushing one's teeth with prussic acid.

How Not To Prevent or Treat an Ingrown Toenail
Many of the myths concerning ingrown toenails revolve around how nails ought to be cut.

I have had many patients tell me that they had been told by the mysterious "they" that if they cut an ingrown toenail in a "V" shape in the middle, their problems would be solved. The reasoning behind this idea is that an ingrown nail is too big, hence if a "V" is cut in the middle, the ends will grow towards the mid-line of the toe, and not into the sides of the nail wall. Unfortunately, this is utter nonsense. You can cut flower patterns out of your toenails, and they will still grow inward if they are incurvated.

One elderly female patient of mine recently told me about her own home remedy for ingrown toenails. Hers is a "poldice" consisting of white bread soaked in milk that has been mixed together with eggs and salt. The "poldice" is apparently applied to the offending toe four times daily if it is to be effective. I do not know how frequently my patient was using it on her toe, but when she last came to my office I had to surgically remove her ingrown nail, and place her on an antibiotic to clear up the infection in the area. I suggested to her that in the future she soak her foot in warm salt water and save her "poldice" to make French toast.

The last thing you ought to do is attempt to remove an ingrown nail yourself. I have already cautioned you in previous chapters of the dangers of bathroom surgery. The same warning applies to an ingrown toenail. If you butcher the job—and the odds are good that you will—you will still have the spicule stuck under the fold of the skin, and you may develop a very nasty infection—if one does not already exist.

Conservative Home Care

One old treatment that does have some merit is the packing of the nail groove with cotton (see Diagram 10:3). With this procedure, the nail is lifted up somewhat from the nail bed, and the nail may then actually grow straight out rather than into the nail wall. However, the chances of success are not that great; there are other treatments that are preferable. But these treatments involve a visit to the doctor's office.

DIAGRAM 10:3
Packing of a Nail Groove

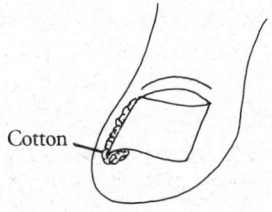

Cotton

Surgery

Before I describe modern surgical techniques for removing an ingrown toenail, I must advise you to avoid an old surgical method that is rather unpleasant. In the bad old days (and no doubt there are still a few doctors around who may use this procedure, hence the warning), the offending part of the nail was excised and the nail-growing plate itself was scraped right down to the toe-bone to prevent regrowth of the incurvation. As you can imagine, this is an uncomfortable experience for the patient, who is incapacitated for a week to ten days after the surgery. Naturally, the risk for post-operative infection is also fairly high with such a procedure.

But there are painless podiatrists, and ingrown nails can be effectively treated with relatively painless "closed" surgery techniques. The primary method is known as *phenol-and-alcohol*—the phenol being an eighty-per-cent-carbolic-acid solution that is used to kill offending plate-growth cells, and the alcohol the disinfectant that prevents the growth of a bacterial infection in the area of the surgery.

The first thing done in the phenol-and-alcohol procedure is to freeze the toe with a local anesthetic. Once the anesthetic has taken hold, the offending part of the ingrown nail is removed with a surgical instrument. Then the nail-growing cells of the part of the nail that is incurvated are destroyed with the application of the phenol to the nail bed. I can assure you that the entire procedure takes only a few minutes, and that the patient is ambulatory immediately after the operation. Very few patients experience more than a mild throbbing in the area even after the anesthetic has worn off. About five per cent of all the patients from whom I have removed ingrown toenails required a few mild analgesic tablets to relieve minor discomfort the first few hours after the surgery. I have never had to prescribe a strong pain-killer for any of those patients who required an analgesic.

There is little post-operative care required as a result of this M.I.S. technique, other than a three-times-daily soaking of the area with warm water and salt for about a week. Because no suturing is necessary, there are no stitches to remove. The procedure is ninety-nine-per-cent effective. However, if there does happen to be a regrowth of a spicule into the side of the nail wall, it will generally occur from twelve to eighteen months after the surgery. The new growth can easily be removed using the same phenol-and-alcohol procedure.

One of the major advantages of the phenol-and-alcohol procedure is that the risk of infection is very low. As a result, people with circulatory problems in their lower limbs, such as diabetics, need not fear the surgical removal of an ingrown toenail any longer.

Moreover, the healing time is much quicker than with old surgical techniques. I have known more than one person who had circulatory problems and ingrown toenails so painful that their life-styles were adversely affected. In fact, a few had become candidates for amputation of the offending toe. Fortunately, this drastic step is no longer considered, since the risk of infection with M.I.S. is less than one half a per cent. The only people who have had the phenol-and-alcohol surgery and have come down with an infection in the area have been those who refuse to obey the rules of post-operative care. The toe must be soaked at regular intervals *until the area has healed*.

There is now a new twist to the phenol-and-alcohol technique. The phenol is replaced by a sodium-hydroxide solution. The advantage of switching to sodium hydroxide is that it takes about a tenth of the time the phenol takes to apply—about fifteen seconds. It is a fairly new development, but I suspect that it will become the norm in the near future.

More Laser Surgery

Laser beams are now being used to remove nail-growth cells. Instead of the application of phenol or sodium hydroxide after an ingrown toenail has been removed, a laser is used to vaporize the nail-growth cells to prevent regrowth of the incurvation. It is thought that there is less trauma to the area, and even less discomfort to the patient, with the use of the laser beam. I imagine that once the equipment becomes less expensive to purchase, the laser technique will probably replace the use of chemicals to destroy the offending nail-growth cells. However, that day is still a bit off in the future.

Rusty Nails

Seventy-five per cent of all the patients I see who are over the age of fifty have at least one fungal nail. These *mycotic* nails—the condition is called in medicalese *onychomycosis*—are really not as bad as they sound, nor are they solely the result of growing old and rusty. However, it seems to be a medical fact that the older you get, the more likely you are to suffer from this disorder, perhaps because a lifetime of neglect of the feet has made you more susceptible. But athletes are also prone to mycotic nails, as you will discover in Chapter Fourteen. So, if you are over fifty, do not feel that you alone are going to be plagued by the problem.

Mycotic nails are caused by a tiny microbe, a fungus, that requires a dark, moist, fairly hot place in which to flourish. The foot fills the bill perfectly, particularly when one is wearing shoes for a long time and perspires freely. Of course, there must be an added ingredient that enables the fungus to settle into a cozy place and grow vigorously to the point at which it becomes noticeable. That ingredient is a handy supply of fresh blood, under the nail, that has been brought to the surface of the nail bed by some sort of injury to the toe. Given a moist, warm, dark spot and a tiny supply of fresh blood, the fungus (*trichophyton rubrum*) will begin to grow, much as any fungus will grow in a mildewy area like a damp towel. It will eventually show up on the nail as a yellowish discoloration.

(Incidentally, athlete's foot is caused by a fungus, as you well know. But, since it is a dermatological problem rather than a nail disorder, I discussed it in the previous chapter.)

The discoloration of the fungal nail can take up to three to four years to become noticeable. At that time the infected part of the nail will appear to detach itself from the nail bed. But even then it may not cause any significant discomfort.

Treating Fungal Nails

Of course there have to be a few old wives' tales about the treatment of fungal nails. I have heard about people with the disorder who have soaked their toes in chlorine detergent, or in a mix of vinegar and water, in a solution of bleach and laundry detergent, and various similar combinations. None of the above will work a permanent miracle. In fact, all the sufferer will probably wind up with is a clean yellow fungus. You will not have to worry where the yellow went; it will still be there.

If you wish to prevent the occurrence of a fungal nail, good hygiene is a must. If you are unlucky enough to injure a toe, a prophylactic application of an anti-fungal cream or powder is advisable.

Once a fungal nail has been definitely diagnosed, treatment that is relatively simple, painless, and efficient can begin.

If the infection is mild, a topical anti-fungal cream is applied to the affected area two or three times daily for a period of a few weeks. Fungi usually grow slowly, but they also take a long time to destroy completely. Therefore, one must be patient. Fortunately, fungal nails are not generally too uncomfortable, so the wait is not that traumatic.

If the fungus has become more obstinate, a stronger cream will work in about sixty per cent of the cases, though it usually works only if one nail is involved. These more potent creams are not readily available over-the-counter, so they will have to be prescribed by a doctor. In the forty per cent of the cases that fail, the foot specialist must proceed to step two.

If topical creams will not eliminate the fungus, the infected part of the nail will have to be excised. As you already know from our discussion of ingrown toenails, this is no longer a major procedure. It is done in the doctor's office under a local anesthetic, and is relatively painless post-operatively. Providing the follow-up use of an anti-fungal cream is continued until the area is completely healed and free of any signs of fungal infection, the success rate for this operation is about eighty per cent.

About twenty per cent of the difficult cases defy both topical cream treatment and excision of the offending nail. If the patient is not experiencing any discomfort worth complaining about, I suggest leaving the nail alone. However, if the fungal nail is causing sufficient pain to warrant further treatment, I will surgically remove the nail and destroy the nail-growing cells (the nail matrix), using the same procedure as I use for the removal of ingrown nails. The advantage of this phenol-and-alcohol surgery is that any incurvation of the nail caused by the growth of the fungus is also taken care of. But I will not proceed to this mode of treatment unless it is absolutely necessary, since the fungus itself is quite harmless and will not infect the rest of the foot.

There is also another treatment, and it is systemic rather than topical. It is the anti-fungal pill, which has been developed in the last few years to combat systemic fungi, particularly those that infect the lungs. As with most medications taken internally, there are side effects involved with anti-fungal pills. In fact, I consider the side effects of these pills to be so severe that I never prescribe them for toenail fungal infections. If it is suggested that you might need to take these pills, make sure that your doctor explains to you how they can adversely affect your overall health.

According to medical literature, the anti-fungal pill is effective in about ninety per cent of the cases. However, it must be taken regularly for up to eighteen months, since it takes that long for a complete toenail to grow. One patient of mine went through this medicinal routine when she was in the care of another doctor. She had all five toenails on one foot infected by the fungus, and had not responded at all to creams or surgery. Her condition was chronic and painful, so the other doctor put her on the pills, and they worked, although she had a wide variety of discomforting, but not life-threatening, side effects. However, I still hold that, normally, if the nail is badly infected by a fungus, it should be totally removed to allow a fresh start. If that does not do the trick, I would then want to remove the nail-growing cells as well, even though the toes may never look esthetically pleasing to the critical eye.

Finally, let me remind you that if a fungal nail is not painful, but only unpleasant to look at, and has not responded to conservative treatment, learn to live with the condition if you can. If you insist on, or require, more aggressive treatment, again my advice would be to live with one less toenail. In the long run you will be none the worse for wear for having lost a fungal nail.

Crazy Nails

I am not referring here to weird and wonderful nail coverings, but to certain other nail problems that come under the general heading of *onychogryphosis*. This medicalese term is used to describe a thick, distorted nail that has become abnormal for a variety of reasons, most often traumatic injury. A less common cause is the constant wearing for years of shoes that do not fit properly. The problem is one of damage to the nail bed and the nail-growing cells. My theory is that if a normal nail has been injured, the nail plate becomes damaged, and the cells respond by growing a thicker nail to protect the nail-growing area and the nail bed. This is not an accepted medical fact, but I believe that my theory does seem logical.

One of the most common of the distorted, or *gryphotic*, nail problems is the *ram's horn* (see Diagram 10:4). In this case, the nail spirals to one side of the toe and takes on the appearance of a ram's horn. However, there are other crazy shapes that a toenail can take if the toe has been traumatized. In all cases the treatment is roughly the same.

DIAGRAM 10:4
A Ram's-Horn Nail

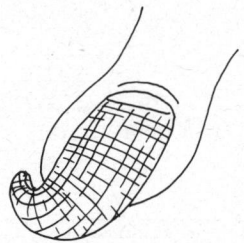

Treating the Crazy Nail

Once the damage has been done, the only treatment that appears to work with any great degree of success is the excision of the entire offending nail using the phenol-and-alcohol technique. However, there are other, more conservative steps that can be tried first. The reason that most people seek relief from gryphotic nails is the same as with fungal nails: they can become painful at times, and they are unpleasant to look at. Yet there are those people who are so embarrassed by the appearance of their distorted toenails that they avoid treatment altogether, even when they are in pain.

The first conservative step I take with those patients who do seek a remedy is to grind, smooth, and trim the gryphotic nail, and have the patient apply moisturizing creams nightly to the affected nail area. The creams will keep the nail soft, and therefore easier to work on.

A concurrent step is to persuade the patient to wear shoes that fit properly. Wearing the proper footwear will relieve pressure on the offending toe and prevent the situation from worsening.

If the deformed nail causes pain, or is too unsightly for the patient to stand, and if conservative treatments do not work, the problem will most likely have to be treated surgically, using the phenol-and-alcohol method. As I mentioned above, this is the only treatment that seems to be quite successful.

The Psoriatic Nail

The psoriatic nail is caused by the presence of *psoriasis* in the skin around the nail, and involves the nail bed where the nail-growing cells are situated.

Psoriatic nails generally become thick and yellow (see Diagram 10:5), and there are often whitish longitudinal lines that run down the nail. A psoriatic toenail will also tend to soften, become brittle, and flake easily.

DIAGRAM 10:5
A Psoriatic Nail

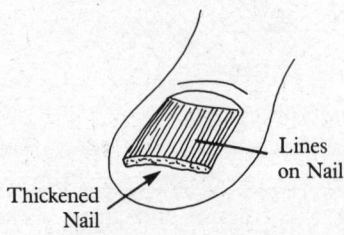

Lines
on Nail

Thickened
Nail

Psoriasis of the nail is most difficult to treat. Some cortisone creams will help a little, but do not offer a permanent cure. Dermatologists at the Psoriatic Research and Education Clinic of Women's College Hospital in Toronto have achieved some success with the application of a coal-tar ointment, along with new experimental drugs that have not as yet been approved for use by the general public.

I hesitate to go into any great detail about treatments, because I believe that anyone with a psoriatic condition, particularly a psoriatic nail, ought to be under a doctor's care rather than be relying on home remedies.

I do not recommend the surgical removal of a psoriatic nail. The reason is that the skin around and under the nail tends to become more prone to psoriasis after nail-removal surgery, and therefore will be more uncomfortable than the affected nail.

Good Nail Hygiene

Now that we have discussed the major nail problems, let us end the chapter by summarizing all the things you can do to keep your nails from causing you trouble.

First, cut your toenails to align with the contour of your toes. If you cut your nails straight across, the jagged edges can catch on things, like socks or pantyhose, and can even irritate adjacent toes. Do not dig out the corners of your nails. You may make them bleed, and that could result in a fungal and/or a bacterial infection. If you do have rough edges on the ends of your toenails, use a nail-file to smooth them.

Try using a mild commercial acid-based preparation that acts to soften the *skin* (not the nail) to prevent an ingrown nail from pushing deep into the skin. A druggist will assist you in the purchase. However, be careful if the nail is incurvated; the acid will not help much, and an overkill of the solution could cause burns and/or infections, just like the indiscriminate use of a corn pad or a callus pad.

If you have been told to soak your toes for a nail problem, I recommend using a saline solution (for example, one teaspoon of Epsom salts to one quart of warm water). If you have a suspected infection in a nail area, and over-the-counter, anti-bacterial or anti-fungal creams or powders do not help, get medical attention quickly to prevent further infection, particularly if the offending area is red, swollen, or discharging.

Bathroom surgery for any condition is, of course, a definite no-no. This applies particularly to anyone with a circulatory problem.

If you injure a toe slightly, and notice some bleeding under the nail, an immediate application of an anti-fungal agent is advisable to prevent a fungal infection. If the nail itself is badly damaged by an accident, I would recommend immediate medical attention to prevent complications, such as those we have discussed in this chapter.

If you have trouble, for whatever reason, cutting your toenails properly, I strongly urge you to have a podiatrist or other foot specialist take care of them for you, or teach you how to care for them properly.

Finally, if you have a circulatory problem to begin with, and develop an abnormal toenail condition, do not play around with the nail yourself—and do not ignore it!

I trust that after having digested all the relevant facts in this chapter, you will now understand why your toenails look like they do, and why you need not fear a trip to the foot specialist to have any abnormalities treated.

11

Systemic Disorders:
INCLUDING CIRCULATORY PROBLEMS, DIABETES, NERVE DISORDERS, GOUT, AND RHEUMATOID ARTHRITIS

Fortunately, as it should be clear by now, most of the foot problems I treat are not systemic; they are biomechanical, and often result in simple wear-and-tear on the lower extremities. However, every body has the means to develop systemic disorders, and these diseases can either directly or indirectly affect the feet.

Out of Circulation

My major reason for concern in patients who could develop systemic foot disorders is poor circulation in the lower limbs. Although I routinely check circulation in a patient's feet, I am particularly careful when the patient is older, is a smoker, is out of shape and/or obese, is a diabetic, or is any combination of the above. I will explain why in a moment.

As far as I am concerned, one of the major detriments to the health of citizens in the so-called "advanced" countries of the world is poor nutrition. It has been clinically shown that a high-fat diet can result in high cholesterol levels in the blood, and that this can translate into cardiovascular disease. The cholesterol, and other fatty acids, will clog arteries as "plaque" that coats the artery walls and thereby narrows the canal through which blood passes (see Diagram 11:1). This disease process is called *atherosclerosis*. When this occurs, there is a lack of proper blood-flow to a given area of the body, particularly to the outer extremities, since they are farthest from the heart, where the fresh, *oxygenated* blood sets out to nourish the body. Because the foot is furthest from the heart, atherosclerotic

160

symptoms will most likely show up first in the feet and lower legs. These symptoms can be quite varied.

DIAGRAM 11:1
Plaque Build-Up in an Artery

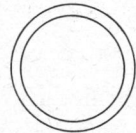 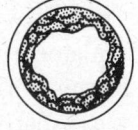

Normal Artery   Plaque Build-Up
in Artery

Reduced blood-flow to a part of the body means that the muscles may become oxygen-deficient. This causes a condition known in medicalese as *intermittent claudication,* a disorder which produces a cramping pain, normally induced by exercise and resulting from an inadequate supply of oxygen to the affected muscles. Usually the muscles in the calf and lower leg are involved. At the same time, the patient's feet may be cold, and it may be difficult to obtain a pulse in the area.

Because exercise—even normal walking—means that the muscles use up more energy than they do when the body is at rest, a person suffering from intermittent claudication will get relief by sitting down and resting until the pain, which can be quite severe, disappears. Many people with this complaint also find that rubbing the affected area helps relieve the pain. In the long run, however, it is best to attend quickly to the circulatory problem that is causing the cramps, rather than just seek temporary relief.

Of course, not all muscle cramps in the legs should be interpreted as a sign of serious cardiovascular disease. However, if you develop the symptoms of intermittent claudication, and your life-style and/ or hereditary predisposition point to potential circulatory disease, you would be wise to seek medical advice immediately.

A person with a circulatory problem in the feet may also develop toenails that are thick and brittle. Hair growth on the lower leg and foot may almost completely cease, and the feet may lose much of their sense of feeling, because of damage to nerves in the area. Therefore, people with circulatory problems will be far more prone than the average individual to frostbite, because they will be unable to tell when their feet are too cold. Poor blood circulation to the feet results in insufficient nourishment to the soft tissues and bones, and therefore greater susceptibility to damage from extreme cold or extreme heat.

In severe cases of circulatory disease, the skin on the foot and lower leg may *ulcerate* because of a serious lack of nutrition to the skin. Unhealthy skin is particularly prone to bacterial infection, and poor blood-flow to that skin means that bacteria-fighting white blood cells will not be available in sufficient quantities to ward off and destroy the bacteria at the site of the infection. Ulcers develop, and the infection becomes even more acute, particularly when a weight-bearing surface of the foot is involved. It is most difficult to treat an ulcerous infection when circulation to the area is impaired, but it is doubly difficult when the wound is continually traumatized by the weight of the body landing on it.

Fortunately there are new treatments to help check and prevent the severe spreading of foot ulcers. These include topical medications, surgical procedures, and even the use of oxygen chambers. *Debriding* (cleansing) agents are used to clean the open wounds by removing foreign material and dead tissue from the area, thereby facilitating the healing process. It is amazing that, not so many years ago, leg and foot ulcers were often incurable, yet it is equally discomforting to note that these ulcers are still a common sight, particularly in much older people who, for whatever reason, are not receiving proper medical attention. Although modern treatment methods have achieved positive results, the best cure for ulcerated feet and legs is still prevention. I would strongly urge those with any circulatory problems to insist that their feet be regularly examined so that any potentially debilitating foot problems can be avoided.

The Diabetic Foot

One of the diseases so often associated with circulatory problems in the lower extremities is *diabetes*. Although this book deals specifically with feet and the lower legs, I should explain a little about diabetes so that you can understand how this disease can adversely affect your feet.

First, let me explain that when I refer to sugar in the bloodstream, I am speaking of *glucose*, which is the sole source of energy for the human brain, and a vital source of nutrition to the rest of the body.

There are basically two types of diabetes. In the first type, the pancreas produces insufficient insulin, which is required to allow sugar to pass from the bloodstream into all the cells of the body. This type of diabetes has been called *juvenile diabetes.* The second form of diabetes is called *mature-onset diabetes* and is more common in adults. It involves the inability of the cells to accept insulin, even though the insulin is being produced by the pancreas in normal, or even increased, amounts. When this happens, the sugar (glucose) levels in the blood increase, and the cells in the body are starved of their energy source.

Before insulin was discovered in the 1920s, people with diabetes did not live very long, since their bodies were being almost entirely robbed of energy. However, thanks to a proper diet, and sometimes to insulin or to oral medications, people with diabetes can now lead almost normal lives. But diabetes can only be controlled; it has yet to be cured. And because the disease is always present in the diabetic person, it must be treated with the greatest respect. Often, when the disease is controlled, the diabetic thinks he or she has been cured and abandons the regimen which controls the disorder.

Diabetics can have foot problems for two major reasons, neither of which has yet been fully explained to the satisfaction of medical researchers. The two problems are *neuropathic* (affecting the nerves) and circulatory.

Diabetics appear to have a higher percentage of circulatory disorders than the non-diabetic population. Moreover, diabetics who fail to take the proper precautions to control their illness are even more at risk than those who follow a proper regimen of diet and medication. As we discussed above, circulatory disorders often manifest themselves first in the feet, because the lower extremities are farther from the heart than any other part of the body. Therefore, it is vital for all diabetics to be made aware of how the disease can affect their feet, and how they can avoid serious foot problems. I have outlined a prevention program below.

Diabetic neuropathy is as serious as circulatory disease when it relates to the foot. And often these two disorders join forces to make life miserable for the diabetic person.

At this point there are only theories, which attempt to explain why diabetes carries with it the side effect of decreased nerve function. The most widely accepted theory is that diabetics can convert glucose to *sorbitol*, a carbohydrate that is also manufactured commercially to be used by diabetics as an artificial sweetener. This extra sorbitol in the body tends to accumulate around nerves and prevent them from functioning normally. New drugs have been produced, in fact, to prevent the body from converting glucose into sorbitol. Time will tell whether or not this theory has merit; I am not as yet in a position to judge.

Because the nerves in the feet are affected adversely, it is often difficult for a diabetic to sense pain or other discomforts, or to distinguish extremely hot and cold temperatures. When poor circulation is combined with a loss of sensitivity, the result may well be some sort of injury or infection that will develop unnoticed until the diabetic is in such dire straits that he or she cannot help noticing the condition. A diabetic may develop a simple blister on a weight-bearing surface of the foot. That blister may turn into an ulcerated lesion that will be most difficult to treat and heal. Ulcers can also develop beneath calluses, corns, and ingrown toenails. An ingrown nail can easily become infected; when left unattended, that infection can become *gangrenous* (that is, the tissues in the area will die), which may lead to amputation. I do not wish to scare anybody reading this book, yet I cannot stress too strongly the acute complications that can arise from the neglect of a foot infection in a diabetic person.

Because a diabetic—or any other person with a circulatory and/or nerve disorder—can acquire a dangerous infection in a foot without feeling any discomfort, prevention becomes paramount. The list of preventive measures below will help you avoid having to deal with such a serious infection.

1.   Use a file to trim your toenails if you are unable to have them cut professionally. Do not use any sharp object that can cut your foot. It stands to reason that bathroom surgery of any kind is strictly forbidden!

2. Do not wear tight, ill-fitting shoes that can irritate your feet to the point of inflaming them. Some ill-fitting shoes may even cut into your feet and cause the area to become infected. If you have purchased a new pair of shoes, check your feet regularly for the first few days to ensure that they are not causing any damage.

3. Check your feet daily, or have someone look at them if you are unable to, to ensure that no fungal or bacterial infections have erupted.

4. Wear natural-fiber—preferably cotton—socks, because they absorb moisture. Dry feet are less prone to infection and inflammation. Do not wear tight, elasticized socks that will hinder circulation in the lower leg and foot.

5. Before you step into a tub of water, check the temperature with the back of your hand to ensure that the water is not too hot. You may not be able to judge the temperature by stepping in if you have reduced nerve function in your feet. Scalded feet do not heal quickly.

6. As a precautionary measure, you may want to wear support hose (this applies to all people with circulatory problems) to help prevent further damage, and, in fact, to assist venous function in the legs. As a result of poorly functioning veins, feet and ankles will swell and become uncomfortable, particularly since shoes will no longer fit comfortably. However, do not confuse support hose with tight stockings. Support hose will aid circulation in the lower limbs; tight socks will reduce circulation. Naturally, support hose that are too tight for you will not be beneficial.

7. Diabetics who exercise are better able to control their condition than those who lead a sedentary life-style. Circulation in the legs and feet definitely appears to be better in diabetics who exercise. This may be due to an increase in *collateral circulation*, a phenomenon whereby smaller blood vessels enlarge as bigger ones in the area become clogged. The newly enlarged vessels may then take over some of the circulatory workload and keep the muscles and other parts of the foot energized. Collateral circulation seems to develop more frequently, and with better results, in people who are active. It is nature's way of rerouting

traffic from clogged arteries and onto the side streets.

There may be quite a few medical experts who refute these theories. But there are also those who suggest that exercise done properly, and the right diet, may even reverse the clogging of arteries. I hope that the latter theory will prove correct—not just to make me feel good, but for the benefit of all those who suffer from diabetes, and a host of circulatory problems.

So I am advising all of you who are diabetic and/or have circulatory conditions to consult the proper medical specialist about undertaking an exercise program tailored to your physical condition and needs. You need not start running or join an aerobics class; a brisk walk every day will suffice for those unable to do more strenuous exercises. I must emphasize that it is never too late for a diabetic to undertake a proper walking program, even if at first you do suffer from intermittent claudication (muscle cramps in the lower legs). I would suspect that the walks will increase your collateral circulation so that the cramps will eventually disappear. But, please, see your doctor first!

8.   It is a good idea to soak your feet daily in lukewarm water and then apply a moisturizing cream. The daily dunking will help keep your feet clean, and therefore less prone to infection. The cream will keep your skin from becoming too dry and cracked, and therefore less prone to infection and inflammation. Also, this daily routine will force you to look at and touch your feet. The daily examination will help prevent any nasty condition from establishing a bridgehead from which it will be difficult to dislodge it.

Gout: The Acid Test

Another systemic disorder that affects the foot—in this case the big-toe joint for some unknown reason—is *gout* (*podagra*, in medicalese, when it refers specifically to the foot).

If you are unlucky enough to suffer from gout, do not feel too badly. Some of the most famous people of all time were fellow sufferers, and in medical dark ages when there was no known treatment for the disease. Their respective gods were not kind to Alexander the Great, Charlemagne, Michelangelo, Martin Luther, Calvin, and

Charles Darwin. It is not inconceivable that Michelangelo would not have been able to translate certain negative emotions to canvas without having suffered terribly from gout. And Calvin might have been a bit less severe had he not suffered from the disease.

Gout, or gouty arthritis, is the end result of a build-up of uric acid in the blood. The uric acid tends to crystallize and settle in joints in the body, most often in the big-toe joint. When it does so, it produces excruciating pain that is often mistaken for a non-disease—osteoarthritis.

Gout is often considered to be a disease of the rich, because in the past only rich people were able to afford tasty diets rich in fatty foods. However, it now appears that while a "rich" diet will exacerbate a gouty condition, the initial problem lies with the body's inability to properly break down the uric acid. In fact, recent studies have led to a theory that uric acid is not a totally useless substance in the body. It may, in fact, aid the body's immune and endocrine systems. We may no longer be able to identify the typical gouty individual as a man of means, sitting at a fully laden dinner table, with grease dripping down onto his royal robes, and one foot with a hugely swollen big toe resting gingerly on a stool beside his chair.

The onset of an attack of gout can be sudden and vicious. It is not uncommon for the victim to be awakened by the excruciating pain in the big-toe joint in the middle of the night. This unexpected, terrible pain distinguishes gouty arthritis from any other form of arthritis. Osteoarthritis, the most common type by far, is characterized by a much slower onset of the condition, chronic pain, and a worsening of the discomfort after a person has been walking or running. Yet despite the differences, it never ceases to amaze me how often the two conditions are mis-diagnosed. Actually, a simple blood test to measure the amount of uric acid in the blood will determine in most cases whether or not the patient has gout.

If gout is not treated properly, it will eventually cause permanent changes in the big-toe joint. The wear-and-tear may necessitate some form of invasive treatment to deal with the breakdown in the joint. Fortunately, there is no need for the disease to ever progress to that stage.

Once the existence of gout has been confirmed, drugs can be prescribed that will control the uric-acid level in the blood. Also, non-steroidal anti-inflammatory drugs can be taken orally to relieve the inflammation in the joint. While gout is definitely not a life-threatening disease, it is indeed a painful one. However, there is absolutely no need for a person to suffer from gout in this day and age.

Rheumatoid Arthritis

Unfortunately, rheumatoid arthritis is a disease that has yet to be tamed. And although it is rarely life-threatening, it can drive a person insane at times because of the relentless pain.

Unlike osteoarthritis, rheumatoid arthritis can affect all age groups, because it is not brought on by a wear-and-tear process. I have seen two-year-olds with the disease. It is thought to be an *auto-immune* condition in which the body's own immune system mistakes the joints for foreign matter, and attacks the joints to destroy them. It is an apparent example of nature at its worst.

Usually, all I can do for a patient with rheumatoid arthritis is provide relief for painful joints in the feet and ankles. I will recommend custom-made shoes and soft supplemental inserts to take much of the normal weight off the diseased metatarsal heads.

If you suspect that you may suffer from this disease, a detailed physical examination and blood tests can determine whether or not you actually do have it. It is important that this disease be treated by a rheumatologist, a specialist well versed in the various diagnostic methods and treatments. Gold or cortisone injections may help alleviate the discomfort, but they do not cure the disease. The same applies for non-steroidal anti-inflammatory drugs taken orally. Modern surgical advances have made the total replacement of some joints possible, but this is done only when the distortion of the joint and the pain no longer allow the patient to function with any degree of normalcy.

Other Systemic Forms of Arthritis

There are other forms of arthritis, and arthritic-type conditions, that can affect the joints of the feet and the lower legs. In fact, there are approximately eighty of them. I have already covered some of them in other chapters; a few are quite rare and are hardly ever seen by foot specialists. Two of those that I do come across from time to time are *psoriatic arthritis* and *gonococcal arthritis*. The latter is caused by the spread of gonococcal bacteria into the joints. I discussed psoriatic arthritis in Chapter Nine; there is little I can say about arthritis brought about by an untreated venereal disease. The symptoms of gonococcal arthritis are similar to any other type of arthritis, but the treatment is basically antibiotic medication to kill the infection.

Neuromuscular Diseases

It would take a large volume to describe in any detail the various diseases that affect the nerves and/or muscles of the lower limbs. These "motor" diseases affect the ability of the lower extremities to move normally. But, because they are usually diagnosed long before I would ever get to examine the patient's feet, there is no point in my getting involved in lengthy descriptions that might only unduly worry or confuse the reader.

I would be remiss, however, if I did not devote a few paragraphs to a discussion of the better-known neuromuscular diseases as they affect the feet and legs. But keep in mind that I am a podiatrist, and therefore not an expert in the diagnosis and treatment of these debilitating disorders.

Until the mid-1950s, when Doctors Salk and Sabin gave the world anti-polio vaccines, *poliomyelitis* was one of the most dreaded of all neuromuscular diseases. Unfortunately, there are many people limping around today who were unlucky enough to contract polio before it was conquered. They were left with at least partial paralysis in one leg, because their motor systems were irreparably damaged.

Polio is now under control almost around the world, but there are numerous other neuromuscular diseases that have to date defied medical researchers. Although the researchers realize that the disorders are caused by a major breakdown of the nervous system, they do not yet understand why this breakdown occurs. As a result, prevention and cures are probably still years away. The diseases we hear about the most in this category are *multiple sclerosis* and *amyotrophic lateral sclerosis* (Lou Gehrig's disease). Both these dreaded diseases eventually rob a person of the ability to use his or her legs and feet.

The Pregnant Foot

Although pregnancy can hardly be classifed as a disease, a pregnant woman's system undergoes changes, most of them hormonal. These changes can affect her feet, particularly as she nears her delivery date and is at her heaviest. All that extra weight puts added stress on her feet, especially when she is walking.

When a woman is pregnant, her ligaments become fairly lax, so that they can expand in order to provide space for the fetus. All the ligaments expand, not just those in and around her stomach and pelvic area. As the ligaments in her feet lengthen, her foot naturally becomes wider and flatter. There is good reason for this: the broader, flatter foot helps distribute the extra weight she is carrying. After a woman delivers, her feet should gradually return to their normal shape, although it is not uncommon for post-partum women to complain that their feet have become permanently enlarged. There is nothing wrong with this situation—as long as the woman buys shoes that fit her new foot size.

I have a bit of advice for the pregnant woman to help her survive the nine months without constantly aching feet and legs. First, wear the proper footwear! I strongly recommend wearing running-shoes with excellent support as much as possible. They provide the best shock-absorption; and you can loosen the laces as the day progresses and your feet begin to swell.

Secondly, your feet begin to swell because the veins in your legs empty into your pelvic area—an area that is being cramped by the normal distension of the womb. As a result, the blood in the veins in the legs backs up because of the traffic jam in the pelvic region, and the feet and legs swell. The two best ways to alleviate the situation are to wear properly fitting support hose—remember, not those that are tight!—and to keep your feet elevated as much as possible.

Finally, if you do have an abnormal pronation problem, it will become more pronounced when you are pregnant because of the change in the shape of your foot. Therefore, you will want to control the abnormal pronation syndrome during your pregnancy, because you will be much more comfortable if you are walking normally, rather than with a biomechanical fault.

Although I advise prevention in almost all cases of biomechanical foot problems, how could I object to motherhood? Yet my mother has constantly reminded me that all her foot problems began after I was conceived. I try to tell her, and all my pregnant patients, that if they follow the advice I give them, they will most likely have perfectly normal feet within weeks of delivering. If only they believed me.

Varicose Veins: In Need of a Valve Job
Pregnant women are obviously not the only people to suffer from poor venous function in the lower limbs. However, it is not abnormal for veins in the legs and feet to perform less than adequately for reasons that have little to do with any specific, serious circulatory condition. Therefore, I have not lumped the discussion of veins and their problems with other circulatory diseases.

I am sure that we all know somebody who suffers, or may have suffered ourselves, from *varicose veins* (as one of my older Eastern European patients once called them, " 'very close veins', because you can see them so close to the skin").

DIAGRAM 11:2
Valves in Veins

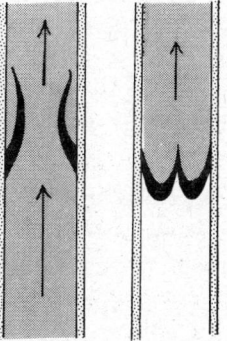

Direction of Blood-Flow   Direction of Blood-Flow

Open Valve   Closed Valve

Varicose veins are veins that have valve problems. As you can see from Diagram 11:2, veins have valves that open to allow blood to pass through and then close to prevent it from flowing backward. This opening and closing action is designed to return spent blood to the heart for passage to the lungs to be re-oxygenated. Unlike the arteries, which carry fresh blood to the various parts of the body, the veins have no muscle fibers to pump the blood. Therefore, the valves are needed to assist the blood-flow back to the heart. Obesity, pregnancy, and overall poor venous function can contribute to the valves malfunctioning. When that happens, blood begins to back up in the veins because it is no longer being forced upwards.

This condition normally affects the superficial veins in the lower leg, particularly on the back or side. These veins expand, because of the blood they are being forced to hold, until eventually they do not function properly. The larger, deeper veins develop valve problems, and at that point the used blood reroutes through smaller, more superficial, veins nearby. These veins are not designed to carry this amount of blood, and they begin to bulge. Unfortunately, the person with varicose veins will often be left with the blues, because the veins usually affected are close to the surface of the skin, and their blue outlines can become quite noticeable. Also, during the time that pressure is building up in these veins, a person can experience quite a bit of pain, often to the point where invasive treatment is required.

There are a number of reasons why people develop varicose veins, and I have already mentioned a few: obesity, pregnancy, and poor valve function. Some people may be victims of their work environments. People who spend long hours every day standing in one spot put tremendous pressure on their legs. Eventually, as the muscles tighten and the areas through which the veins must pass become impeded, the excess strain affects the circulation. Deoxygenated blood gets backed up in the veins, which can then swell and eventually develop valve problems. As I mentioned above, pregnant women can also be victims, although the problem arises from poor venous function in the pelvic area rather than in the lower legs themselves.

If you discover that you are developing varicose veins, what can you do to relieve the symptoms and prevent the situation from deteriotating? First, you ought to change your work habits as much as possible, so that you are not standing in one spot for long periods of time. Secondly, you should wear support hose, because, as I previously mentioned, they help venous function.

If you have painful varicose veins, and/or you wish to do something to improve your appearance cosmetically, you could undergo surgery to remove or collapse the veins. The blood will naturally find its way into veins nearby.

A Swell Time
Many people complain of swollen feet and ankles when they have been sitting or standing in one place for a long time, particularly in hot, muggy conditions. Unless they have an already diagnosed circulatory problem, they should not worry too much, because this is a normal phenomenon.

Because most people complain of this problem during long airplane flights, a misconception has developed that the atmosphere in the plane is the cause. But it is actually the sitting position that is to blame. When your legs are bent at the knees, the area through which the blood flows back through the veins is cramped, and your circulatory system in your lower extremities is adversely affected. Therefore, normal venous function is disrupted temporarily. The obvious solution is to walk around as much as possible during the flight to allow the lower limbs to stretch out and to increase the space through which the veins must pass. Or, if you are lucky enough to be on a fairly empty plane, put up your feet and relax. The law of gravity will take care of the venous function in your legs.

The Demon Rum and the Evil Weed
I have seen so many patients who shrink at the thought of poisoning themselves with any type of medication, but who think nothing of the toxicity of the cigarettes they smoke or the excessive amounts of alcohol they consume. Although these people have a right to be concerned about the potentially dangerous side effects of certain drugs, they ought to be aware of what excessive alcohol and smoking can do to them.

Before we speak of alcohol and tobacco specifically, I must define two terms for you. The first is *vasodilation*, and it refers to a temporary expansion of a blood vessel. Heat is an example of a *vasodilator*, as are a number of drugs and other chemicals we ingest or inject. *Vasoconstriction* is the opposite of vasodilation, and can be caused by cold, or by a variety of drugs and other chemicals. Tobacco is a well-known *vasoconstrictor*. Keep in mind then that vasodilators work to increase blood flow through the circulatory system;

vasoconstrictors act to decrease blood flow through the circulatory system, and this decrease could become acute and/or chronic.

There is little doubt in medical circles today that not only can smoking damage the lungs, but it can also contribute greatly to cardio-vascular disease that can have effects on the feet. I join with cardio-vascular specialists in strongly urging my patients with systemic foot conditions to quit smoking. I know of many vascular surgeons who absolutely refuse to operate on patients who will not, or cannot, quit smoking. Naturally we doctors do not confine our advice to those who are already ill. An ounce of prevention is worth much more than just a pound of cure. Quitting smoking will keep you on your feet, and healthier, for a lot longer than if you continue to puff away.

As for the "demon rum", it is not supposedly that bad for you from a medical standpoint, if consumed in small "medicinal" amounts. Studies have indicated that small quantities of alcohol may act as vasodilators, and can therefore improve blood-flow for a couple of hours for people with circulatory problems.

However, the consumption of large amounts of alcohol over a long period of time is destructive to the human body, as we all know. Many addictive drinkers first show signs of *alcoholic neuropathy* in their legs and feet. This means that nerve function in their lower limbs has been affected as the accumulative effects of the consump-tion of large quantities of alcohol attack the central nervous system. So, if you like to tipple and begin to experience pins and needles, numbness, and loss of sensation in your feet, you would be wise to seek a medical opinion at once. You may be on the verge of self-destructing.

There may be other recreational drugs and medications that adversely affect the lower extremities, but it would take a few volumes to cover all the potential risks. I would suggest that if you are at all concerned about the side effects of certain drugs or other products you may be ingesting, you ought to consult with your family physician, or other qualified expert, on the toxicity of various medications, recreational drugs, and such things as food additives.

Cold Comfort
Before discussing serious problems like immersion foot (chilblain)

and frostbite, I would like to clear up a couple of misconceptions.

First, there is absolutely no connection between having so-called "cold feet" and being afraid to do something. Your extremities do not necessarily drop in temperature when you have fears about making a major decision. Secondly, if you get your feet wet, you are no more likely to catch cold than if you were perfectly dry. If you leave your feet sitting in cold water long enough, you may eventually cause some damage to them, but you will not suddenly develop all the symptoms of a viral infection.

Immersion Foot, or Chilblain

Immersion foot, or *chilblain*, is probably the most common cold-related injury to affect the feet. It can occur in temperatures as high as 15°C (60°F) and as low as freezing (0°C or 32°F), or even lower. A damp environment, particularly that inside a wet shoe, is often a contributing condition. Immersion foot most commonly affects those with poor circulation, particularly women who wear tight-fitting shoes that reduce circulation to the forefoot.

Symptoms of immersion foot include a whitish color in the affected area, some swelling (*edema*) caused by the build-up of protective fluid under the skin, blistering from the edema, itching, and some pain. However, the affected part of the foot is not frozen.

The treatment is relatively uncomplicated. Analgesics may be required for a few days to relieve pain in the affected area. Whirlpool baths may help increase circulation in the feet. A change in footwear may also be necessary. Care must be taken to ensure that blisters do not break and become infected. Because the disorder can recur quite easily in the proper conditions, it is advisable to avoid cold, damp weather whenever possible. If you must be out in fairly inclement weather, you could wear two pairs of socks to better insulate your feet. Wool socks trap the most heat to keep your feet warm. Silk is not bad, if you can afford silk socks, and certain types of padding and liners can also help keep the feet warm and dry. If you are active and out in cold weather, try not to wear cotton socks, because cotton absorbs too much moisture and dries slowly. Also, its ability to trap and hold warm air in between its fibers is not as good as other fabrics.

Frostbite

Frostbite is far more serious than immersion foot. It may be quite superficial and involve only the outermost layers of the skin, or it can penetrate the entire foot to the point at which the only treatment is amputation of the foot to prevent the spread of gangrene.

In frostbitten areas the blood, nerve, and soft-tissue cells are frozen. If the damage is extensive and deep, it may be permanent. Therefore, the utmost caution must be taken to prevent the onset of frostbite, or, if it has occurred, to treat it quickly and properly.

The symptoms of frostbite vary somewhat from those of immersion foot. The skin initially becomes bluish-white, and there is a burning pain in the affected area. Eventually the skin assumes a waxy appearance, and the victim feels warmth in the area. But the foot will soon become numb and feel very heavy. There will be occasional sensations of tingling along with the numb, heavy feeling.

The best treatment for any degree of frostbite is immediate medical attention. If that is not possible, there are a few steps to avoid and a few to take to minimize the damage to the foot.

First, do not rub the affected part of the foot, especially with something cold, like snow. There is no circulation in the frostbitten area, so rubbing it will accomplish nothing, and the cold snow will only increase the insult. Secondly, do not expose the frostbitten area to extreme heat, such as hot water or a fire. You may accidentally burn already damaged tissue. Thirdly, do not smoke or drink alcohol, because blood-flow to the foot will be decreased further. Fourthly, it is probably wise not to try and walk on the affected foot. I say "probably", because some medical researchers do not believe that this precaution is necessary.

I advise that the affected area be soaked immediately in tepid water, although some experts believe that the water may be warmer, but not hot. Once the entire foot becomes reddish in color—after about twenty minutes if the frostbite is not too severe—it may be removed from the water. Pain in the affected area will probably be acute during the thawing-out process, so it might be advisable to take a strong analgesic. Some frostbite experts also recommend that the victim drink warm liquids, or even a *small* amount of alcohol, after the foot has been soaked, to help increase blood-flow to the feet.

The feet will swell due to the build-up of protective fluid. Therefore, it would be prudent to keep the lower extremities as elevated as possible after the frostbitten area has been removed from the warm water.

Frostbitten parts of the body are more susceptible to bacterial infection than normal tissue. They may also be more prone to fungal infection during the recovery process. It would be wise to ensure that these infections never get a chance to develop. To that end, I repeat that it is vital that proper medical attention be received as soon as possible after the injury has been incurred.

As you might expect, once a part of the foot has been subjected to frostbite, it will be more vulnerable to repeated episodes than will unaffected areas. So you will have to take certain precautions to prevent the recurrence of such an insult. As with the precautions you take to prevent immersion foot, proper footwear—including shoes, inserts, and stockings—must be worn in cold weather. And, if at all possible, a person who has suffered from frostbite should try to avoid being exposed to extremely cold temperatures.

This ends our discussion of foot problems that are caused by systemic diseases. Please keep in mind that these conditions are the exceptions rather than the norm when it comes to podiatric practice. Although I have done my best not to scare you, and have tried to explain all the disorders with a minimum of medicalese, I would suggest that if you had any foot problems that you were worried about because they sounded systemically induced, you would not hesitate to seek immediate medical attention. It is far better to be reassured by a doctor that the problem is not serious than to wander around wondering if your health is in danger.

12

Children's Feet

Starting Off on the Right Foot

I would have to say that some of my most interesting patients are children, not only because they are fascinating subjects who are likely to say and do the nuttiest things while in my office, but also because pediatric foot care (*podopediatrics*) is often a challenging, and very rewarding, experience.

One of the problems with podopediatrics is that there is a lack of genuine research on birth defects of the foot, or on the difference between the normal and the abnormal foot in infants from birth up to the age at which they normally begin to walk (about ten to eighteen months). Another problem has to do with parental misconceptions about infant footwear, and about the development of the lower limbs of a child. A third problem is the inexperience of certain medical professionals in dealing with what could be an infantile foot problem, either because they do not consider the foot to be all that important compared to the rest of the baby's body, or because they have never learned enough about podopediatrics in the first place to recognize a problem until it becomes blatantly obvious.

Before we look at specific foot problems affecting infants, it might be wise to differentiate between the normal and the abnormal foot, during the growth of the limbs in the womb and then from birth on.

Thanks to the wonders of modern photographic techniques and space-age technology, it has been possible to show that the *limb buds*—the beginnings of the arms and legs—start to form about four weeks after conception. One week later it should be possible to recognize the shape of the foot. By the twenty-sixth week, the embryonic foot should be fully developed. At birth a normal infant, after a normal delivery, ought to have fully developed feet with all the soft-tissue formations, nerves, and circulatory system in place. All the bones are also present at birth, with the exception of the two end bones (the *distal phalanges*) of the baby toes. Naturally, the standard model will include five toes on each foot, complete with minuscule toenails. All the bones in the infant's foot undergo changes in size, shape, and position as the foot prepares itself for weight-bearing.

When a doctor is examining a newborn baby to determine whether or not the feet are normal in all respects, he or she must consider the lower limbs as complete units. It is vital to check the positioning of the foot vis-à-vis the overall shape of the leg and the positions of the hips and knees. Potential problems exist if the baby is decidedly *bow-legged* or *knock-kneed* (see Diagram 12:1). If these problems exist, the foot of the child will be affected, particularly as it begins to walk, and especially if the infant's legs are twisting internally or externally (*internal* or *external torsion*) at the same time.

DIAGRAM 12:1
Abnormal Lower-Limb Positions in Children

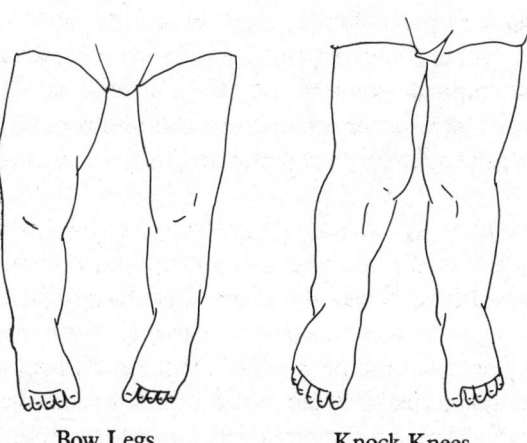

Bow Legs   Knock Knees

After I examine the lower limbs as a whole, I turn my attention to the feet themselves. Because of the many intricate motions of the foot and ankle, it is not easy for a practitioner to tell the normal from the abnormal, and I am therefore very exacting in my manipulations. However, I must assure you that, according to the most recent statistics, only one infant in a hundred who is a full-term baby and has had an uneventful delivery will suffer from an abnormal foot problem that will require immediate attention.

I always stress to new parents with babies who have normal feet that their children ought to be left alone to develop by themselves. Also, since getting back to nature seems to be one of the themes of the present decade, I tell these anxious parents what my pediatrics professor told me back in medical school many years ago.

"If God in his infinite wisdom," he said, "had meant babies to wear shoes, they would have been born with them." The only function of the shoe as far as pre-walkers are concerned is to keep their feet warm when necessary. There are cheaper ways to keep an infant's feet warm. The only other thing shoes can do for an infant who is not yet walking is to harm the feet if they are ill-fitting. So, unless you are really anxious to get that first pair of shoes bronzed, I would advise you to save your money until baby actually needs the footwear to protect his or her feet.

I also advise parents not to play around with their infant's feet. If they suspect that their baby has a foot deformity or a lesser problem, they would be well advised to seek an opinion from a podopediatrist or an orthopedic surgeon who specializes in children's foot disorders. There is a very high success rate in the conservative treatment of the usual range of infantile foot disorders, if the problem is identified and dealt with at the outset, before the abnormality has had a chance to develop further.

The Club Foot

The number-one fear that expectant parents have about the feet of the baby is that it will have a *club-foot* deformity (*talipes equinovarus*, in medicalese). A club foot is usually twisted downwards and inwards, although there are variations in which it is twisted outward (*talipes valgus*), or in which just the sole of the foot is turned inwards (*talipes varus*) (see Diagram 12:2). Obviously, unless such a birth defect is corrected immediately, the baby will have a tough time walking normally when it begins to try getting up off all fours.

DIAGRAM 12:2
The Club Foot in Children

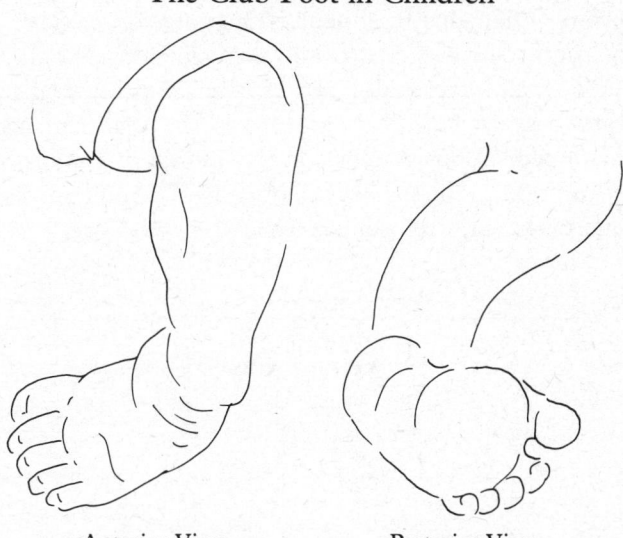

Anterior View   Posterior View

The club foot is a birth defect, which was thought to be caused by the abnormal position of the fetus in the womb during the gestation period. This theory held that there was no particular reason why the normal development of the lower limbs was affected during pregnancy; the unborn child just happened to be positioned in the wrong place for too long a time, and the foot did not have the space in the womb to grow in the proper direction. According to the recent medical literature on the subject, the position has little to do with club feet. It holds that the ankle bone develops abnormally, and causes a dislocation between it and the navicular, which in turn creates further bone and soft-tissue problems during development of the fetus.

A club foot is easily recognizable at birth, so there is no reason to delay treatment. In fact, my old professor of podopediatrics used to say that he wished babies born with a club foot would emerge feet first so that he could begin treatment more quickly. The treatment of choice in mild cases is to place the offending foot and lower leg in a plaster cast, thereby forcing the limb to assume a more normal position. To ensure proper development as the infant grows, the cast is either changed or "wedged" every couple of weeks. As you can see from Diagram 12:3, a wedged cast has a pie-shaped inversion cut out of it to provide extra space for the rapidly developing lower limb to grow. When this treatment is begun at once, there is little reason for more radical steps to be taken down the road, and the infant's foot should eventually develop well within normal limits. In moderate-to-severe club-foot deformities, the treatment, according to many orthopedists, ought to be corrective surgery, performed early in infancy to prevent abnormal development. I am inclined to agree with them after having seen some excellent results.

DIAGRAM 12:3
A Wedged Cast

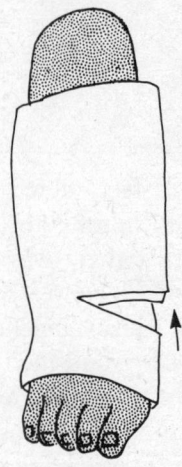

In milder cases, the limb will be in a cast for from ten to twenty-six weeks, depending on the severity of the club foot. Therefore, the shape of the foot ought to be within acceptable limits long before the infant is ready to take his or her first steps.

It is important that complete X-ray evaluation and other follow-up examinations be conducted on a regular basis after the cast has been removed to ensure that all the bones of the foot and lower leg are present and are growing in the right directions. These follow-up examinations should be conducted for the first two years of the child's life to make sure that there is no regression. It is sometimes necessary during that period to place the child in a *straight-lasted* shoe (see Diagram 12:4) that will help maintain the correction during the early development of the foot.

DIAGRAM 12:4
The Dennis-Browne Bar

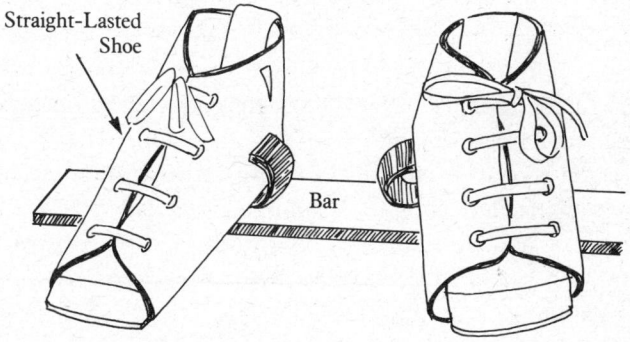

Straight-Lasted Shoe

Bar

Other Congenital Problems

There are a few other concerns arising from poor positioning of the unborn child in the womb. One of those is called *metatarsus adductus*, which is medicalese for the front part of the foot turning inwards at birth. The opposite, outward, turning is also possible, but far less common. This is a condition of the metatarsal bones only. If the first metatarsal only is involved, the condition is called *metatarsus primus adductus* or *varus*. As with the club foot, metatarsus adductus is not common in newborn babies, and is readily treatable, particularly if the condition is dealt with from the beginning of the infant's life.

Both metatarsus adductus and metatarsus primus adductus are easily noticed by the trained eye, although when the conditions are very mild they will not be seen until the child begins to walk. However, mild cases respond well to treatment, even if not caught at birth.

If either condition is severe enough, it may be necessary to put the offending foot in a plaster cast for the first few weeks of the baby's life. Thereafter—and in most milder cases—it is advised to place the infants in reversed straight-lasted shoes fastened together by a *Dennis-Browne bar* or a *Brachman skate* (also Diagram 12:4) whenever necessary. These contraptions are worn while the child is asleep to keep the feet properly positioned at all times. It is also important to remember that orthotics may be required to maintain the correction once it has been made.

If properly treated during the early growth period of the child, both metatarsus adductus and metatarsus primus adductus respond exceptionally well, and the infant will be able to stand and walk normally when the time comes.

Another condition that occasionally crops up with newborn infants, and causes a lot more concern to parents and ogling grandparents than it merits, is *overlapping*, or *curled*, toes. One of the ironies of my profession is that my middle child was born with an overlapping toe. The pediatrician who first examined my daughter was highly amused that a podiatrist could help produce a child with such a condition.

An overlapping toe is not a serious deformity problem. Many of them will automatically straighten out by themselves, but a few will have to be taped to adjacent toes for a few months to keep them permanently in line. During this time there is no discomfort to the infant, only to the concerned family and friends. By the time the infant is ready to get up on its feet, the offending toe, or toes, will have straightened out, and the first steps will be just normally awkward, rather than abnormally awkward.

One deformity, however, that is not caused by poor positioning of the fetus in the womb is a condition known as *supernumary toes*, and it is congenital because, for some reason, the developing fetus was doled out more than five toes per foot. Although there have been rare cases in which a newborn baby had more than six toes, I have never seen more than a half-dozen.

Supernumary toes can occur on one foot or both feet. Obviously it is one of the easiest disorders to diagnose; the extra toe is usually found on the outside of either the big toe or the baby toe. Not only is the diagnosis simple, but treatment is also relatively easy.

The extra toe (or toes) can be removed surgically, either immediately after birth, or once the baby is considered strong enough for the operation. A quick fix is not essential for the development of a normal foot, although surgery should be performed as soon as possible before the baby decides to attempt to walk. An early resolution to the problem is recommended when parents and grandparents become obsessed with an offspring's abnormality. In any event, surgery is almost always easy and successful, and perhaps parents of children born with extra toes could consider the occurrence as an omen of extra good fortune, rather than as one of bad luck.

Finally, fewer than one per cent of all newborn babies arrive on the scene with webbed feet. However, this does not mean that they are ugly ducklings doomed to a childhood of woe. What happens is that during the maturation process in the womb, the toes of the fetus are somehow joined together by skin between the interspaces (see Diagram 12:5). As with many minor infantile foot problems, it is the parents or grandparents who clamor for immediate surgery.

DIAGRAM 12:5
Webbed Toes

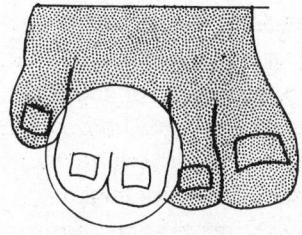

In actual fact, unless X-rays show a bone deformity of some sort, there is no reason to ever detach the joined toes. A child can grow up with attached toes and walk or run quite normally, except when they are completely webbed to the nails. I have seen quite a few adults with webbed feet who have never experienced any dysfunction or discomfort.

However, there are those parents who insist that their baby be relieved at once of the webs. Fortunately, the procedure is quite simple: minor plastic surgery to cut the skin between the toes, and then stitching of the flaps. The infant will experience little real discomfort, and the incisions should heal quickly.

Now that we have covered the most common lower-limb deformities in infants at birth, let us turn our attention to babies beginning to walk.

The Sneaker Generation

I know it may not be quite as appealing to bronze baby's first pair of sneakers for posterity, but that is the type of footwear your offspring ought to be wearing as he or she grows up, because they provide the best sort of support for the normal growing foot at the most reasonable cost. Before I explain exactly why sneakers are the preferred form of footwear for the growing child, I would like to trace the development of the foot from the time the child begins to walk until he or she is fully grown.

The first thing to get perfectly straight is the fact that a child's limbs do not necessarily grow the same amount at the same time. However, by the end of a youngster's physical development, both legs ought to be the same basic length—all things being equal, and give or take a couple of millimeters. So you need not panic if you think that your child is listing as he or she walks and you discover that one leg is a bit shorter than the other.

I have seen cases where children were prescribed shoe-lifts for their shoes because at one given moment one leg was longer than the other, and the end result was a biomechanical problem that would never have occurred once the lower limbs were both naturally fully grown. The moral of the story is not to try and fool with nature, because once it has made adjustments for an artificially produced abnormality, those adjustments will be difficult to completely eliminate without further, and expensive, treatment. It is only in the rare case where the discrepancy in the length of a child's legs is more than a half-inch to three-quarters of an inch that one ought to consider eliminating the difference with special treatment, such as a shoe-lift. And it will be important even then to watch the child's development carefully so that the lifts can be changed or removed completely as the child grows.

Another concern of parents that is often totally unnecessary is that their child is a very late walker. Then, when they realize all the mischief an infant who is walking can get into as compared to one who is still on all fours, they are sorry that the kid ever took that first step. Babies usually begin to walk between the ages of ten and eighteen months. Some take their first steps before this if they have developed early physically and their lower limbs can support them; others wait until they are well over two years of age. Often the late starters are not physically ready to walk, but occasionally they just do not feel the need. My co-writer was two and a half before he took his first steps, and he had to be bribed with candy held for him across the room before he finally got up off all fours.

In-toeing and Out-toeing

When parents come to my office with youngsters who have just begun to walk, their most common complaints are that their offspring are waddling like ducks or taking pigeon-toed steps. Often these unusual gaits result from the infant's attempt to maintain balance on still-unsteady lower limbs, and the child will usually begin to walk properly as the lower limbs develop normally. It is common for newly walking babies to toe out dramatically, and to appear to lack arches altogether. The apparent abnormalities in gait are only nature's way of helping an infant remain erect.

However, if a small child continues to either *toe in* or *toe out* (see Diagram 12:6), there is probably a bone deformity or muscle weakness present in the lower limbs, and the abnormality may have to be corrected. Otherwise the child will continue to grow and to walk abnormally, and will probably be the butt of cruel jokes at school, at play, and even in the home. A child who is constantly being teased about the way he or she walks will not be a happy child.

In-toeing and out-toeing can be spotted in a baby's first steps, and it is often sharp-eyed grandparents who are the first to notice the problem. About sixty-five per cent of the time the child toes in; the rest of the time he or she toes out.

In mild cases of in-toeing or out-toeing, the problem is generally caused by a minor bone deformity or muscle weakness. As with most of the very mild infantile foot disorders, detection at birth

DIAGRAM 12:6
Abnormal Toeing In and Toeing Out in Children

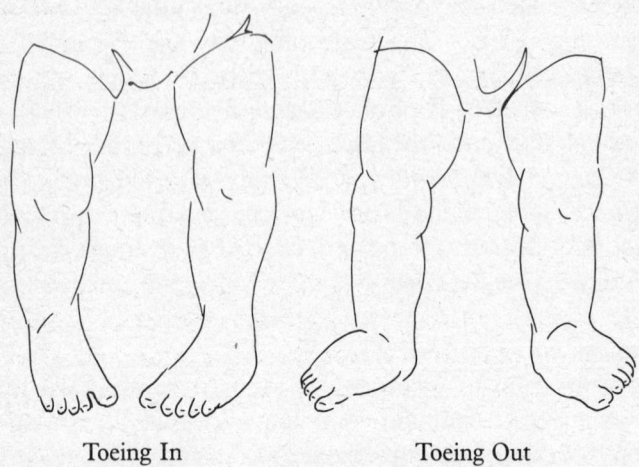

Toeing In   Toeing Out

is not easy, since the foot is shaped normally, although the tilt of the foot will be abnormal. However, this tilt is not usually evident until the baby begins to take steps. My advice to parents who have infants with a mild degree of in-toeing or out-toeing is to leave them alone, because the situation will take care of itself with time. If it becomes obvious after the infant has been walking for a while that a serious in-toeing or out-toeing problem exists, this is an indication of the presence of a more severe bone deformity or muscle weakness. As the problem gets more severe, the treatment must be more aggressive. Rest assured, however, that with proper conservative care your child will not waddle around like a duck or toe in like a pigeon forever.

The normal amount of in-toeing or out-toeing is about 15 degrees. And, as I mentioned above, it is perfectly normal for the arch to appear flat for the first few months that the baby is walking. At this point in the child's development, the arch area is actually filled with "baby" fat that flattens out and cushions the foot and provides better balance and mobility for the child. As the child grows, the arch should develop normally, but if it does not, you ought to consult a specialist for an appraisal of the situation.

However, it has been my experience that ninety-five per cent of the children I see under the age of four who have in-toeing or out-toeing tendencies are within normal limits, and they will eventually outgrow their problems without intervention of any kind.

If a child is toeing out to the point at which medical intervention is required, because of a *tibia* (shinbone) deformity (the condition is known as *external tibial torsion*) or a misalignment at the ankle joint, the usual treatment is wearing the Dennis-Browne bar or the Brachman skate (the same contraptions used to rectify metatarsus adductus) at bedtime. The bar or the skate is attached with the shoes facing inward to realign the foot. It should not be necessary to keep the child in these appliances nightly for more than a few months. The important thing to watch with this treatment is that you do not over-correct the original deformity. Otherwise the child will eventually have to wear the bar or the skate with the shoes facing in the opposite direction when he or she is sleeping at night.

If, for whatever reason, a child is allowed to develop with a definite out-toeing problem, it may be necessary for orthotic devices to be worn for eighteen to twenty-four months to correct the disorder. Older children do not respond well to the wearing of applicances on their feet at night while they sleep.

In-toeing can be caused by metatarsus adductus or *internal tibial torsion*, both of which appear to force the foot to turn to the inside. Children who toe in seem to be perpetually off balance, because they are. It is not easy to walk pigeon-toed and keep one's balance, whatever one's age.

The treatment for in-toeing, if caused by internal tibial torsion or metatarsus adductus, is basically the same as for out-toeing. However, when the Dennis-Browne bar or the Brachman skate is put on, the shoes are pointed outward rather than inward to force the feet to the outside. Also, it may be necessary to place orthotic devices in the child's shoes for up to two years, depending on the severity of the problem. The treatment usually works quite well if the condition is spotted early. If the cause is excess femoral antiversion, which is usually found in three-to-six-year-olds, the "W" sitting position (see Diagram 12:7) is recommended whenever possible.

DIAGRAM 12:7
The "W" Position

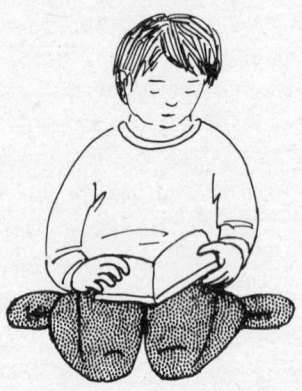

Growing Pains: Problems of Older Children

Children can still toe in or toe out past the age of three if their conditions are ignored or acquired. Treatment of these disorders is not as simple as with toddlers, because older children tend not to lie still at night in Dennis-Browne bars or Brachman skates. Also, they do not seem to respond to straight-lasted shoes. So, what can we do when suddenly concerned parents come rushing into the office with their decidedly knock-kneed, bow-legged, or severely pronating children?

Unfortunately, there are still a few doctors who believe that a child past the age of about eight will outgrow in-toeing or out-toeing. It rarely happens. These children may have to be fitted with orthotics that help realign the foot and lower leg. Orthotics work amazingly well with this age group, and it is always gratifying for me to see a child who first came to me with a severe problem walk normally after a few months of wearing an orthotic device. Of course, there are some cases that take longer to treat successfully, so if your child has been fitted with orthotic devices, and you have yet to see dramatic improvement after a few months, be patient.

Another pain for children from the ages of about five to fifteen is felt directly in the foot. Children who abnormally pronate severely and are allowed to continue to do so will eventually wind up with a bunion. There are two schools of thought when it comes to treating a bunion on a child's foot, and both of them, unfortunately, involve surgery. There is no quick fix for this condition, unless the parents and the child are willing to put up with a lifetime of discomfort, because, even if the pronation problem is corrected, the bunion, once developed, will not magically disappear.

I agree with some of my colleagues who feel that early bunion surgery on a still-developing foot could result in damage to the *growth plate* of the big-toe bone. The long-term result could be a serious bone deformity. Therefore, we prefer to delay bunion surgery until the growth plate has completely united with the big-toe bone.

The other school of thought is that the correction to the big-toe bone ought to be done as quickly as possible, before the child has a fully developed foot. Surgeons who hold this belief argue that they do not touch the growth plate at all. Moreover, the earlier the operation is performed, they say, the less damage there will be to soft tissue around the bony deformity, and the more likely the toe will be to grow in the right direction.

I believe that there is merit in the second argument. However, I still prefer to wait until the growth plate of the big-toe bone has fused with the bone, so that the possibility of damage to the plate no longer exists.

Breaking Up Is Easy To Do
It is hardly uncommon for active children to fracture bones in their limbs. Fortunately, at a young age they tend to heal quickly—usually within four to eight weeks if they are treated properly with a cast to immobilize the fractured bone while it mends.

There is no sense going into details to describe all the possible fractures a child can suffer in a foot, since most of the bones are vulnerable if traumatized severely. But it is important to recognize the symptoms of a break and deliver the child to the proper medical center for X-ray evaluation and immediate treatment. If the child screams in agony when the injured area of the foot is palpated, and if there is considerable swelling accompanying the pain, a fracture has to be considered.

Once the diagnosis has been made and the fractured bone is immobilized, it will be necessary to X-ray the area periodically until the orthopedic surgeon or podiatrist is convinced that the bone has healed in a proper alignment, and that there has been no damage to the growth plate of that bone.

Breaking Down Under Stress

Another common orthopedic condition in children is *aseptic necrosis* of an *epiphysis*. This is a non-infectious breaking down of the growth plate of a bone. The generally accepted theory in medical circles is that the condition is caused by trauma to a given part of a bone while a child is playing hard or engaged in some other strenous activity. In the foot, the most common bones affected are the heel bone, the *navicular* in the midfoot, and the second metatarsal. Because the condition involves the growth plate of the bones, and since that growth plate eventually fuses with the end of its bone as a child reaches his or her late teens, aseptic necrosis of the epiphysis (growth plate) is strictly a childhood disease.

The first example of aseptic necrosis I will discuss is *Freiberg's disease*. If a child constantly complains of pain under the second metatarsal head, especially during or after strenuous activity, there is a decent chance that the growth plate of the metatarsal bone is breaking down. In fact, as you can see in Diagram 12:8, in severe cases the metatarsal head can almost completely disappear. However, the metatarsal head usually regenerates by itself with time, although I have seen many cases where the bone remains abnormally shaped

DIAGRAM 12:8
Freiberg's Disease

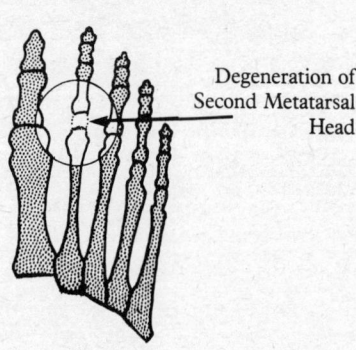

Degeneration of
Second Metatarsal
Head

throughout a person's life. Even if this happens, it would be unusual for the pain to persist after the child has stopped growing. If the area remains painful, I will X-ray the bone to ascertain whether or not it is regenerating properly, but I would advise patience rather than aggressive intervention if the condition persists.

DIAGRAM 12:9
Growth Plate of Heel Bone Affected by Sever's Disease

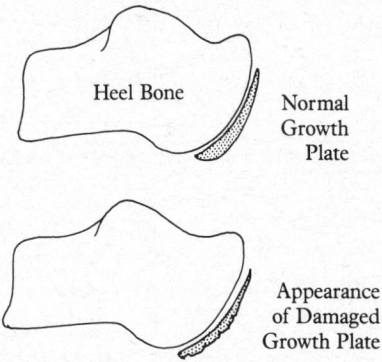

Sever's disease (Diagram 12:9) affects the heel bone of growing, active children—almost always males—and will last until approximately the age of fourteen. The child will complain of a sharp pain in the back of the heel when he or she is playing or running. As with other forms of aseptic necrosis, there is no need to worry excessively about Sever's disease. Once the growth plate fuses solidly to the heel bone, the pain will disappear for good.

The navicular bone is ship-shaped, as you see in Diagram 12:10, and it articulates (combines to form a joint) with the three cuneiform bones in front and with the ankle bone at the back. It is a sturdy part of the anatomy, and is rarely mentioned outside medical circles. However, children can fall victim to aseptic necrosis of the growth plate, and they will complain of pain in the area of the navicular bone. The condition is known as *Kohler's Navicular* or *Kohler's disease* (Diagram 12:10).

DIAGRAM 12:10
Kohler's Navicular

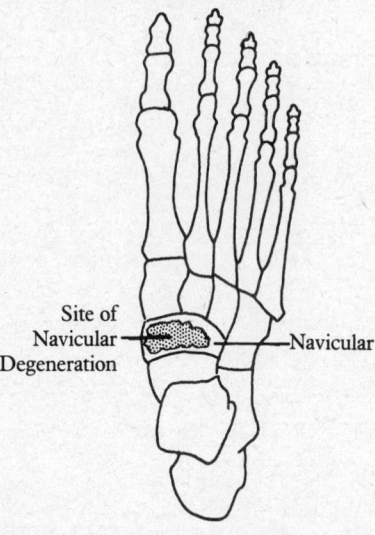

Site of
Navicular —
Degeneration

—Navicular

As I have already mentioned, aseptic necrosis of a growth plate can be confirmed by X-rays. The affected area, when viewed from the side, will appear ratty, or moth-eaten. Of course, there is nothing gnawing away at the growth plate. And, in all cases, natural healing will take place over a period of time, until the growth plate fuses solidly to its bone. Orthotics can be used to relieve pressure to the affected areas if the pain is severe, and they are particularly effective in Freiberg's disease. A remedial arch may lessen the discomfort of Sever's disease and Kohler's disease, and a heel pad may provide relief for Sever's-disease sufferers. However, the shoe inserts do not cure the conditions; nature does, with time. The wearing of proper footwear will also lessen the symptoms; ill-fitting shoes never helped any foot problem. If the pain is particularly acute after strenuous activity, particularly in the heel area, the application of ice can help relieve the inflammation.

If a child suffers from an aseptic necrosis in the foot, a parent may feel it necessary to curtail the offspring's physical activities. Such a drastic step is usually not necessary. The child should be allowed to continue his or her activities up to the point where the discomfort level eclipses the pleasure level. The activities will not permanently damage the foot.

Young Maids' Knees

Some young women, usually between the ages of thirteen and eighteen, experience annoying knee pain, particularly when going up or down stairs, after sitting a long time and then getting up, and intermittently whenever the knee decides to protest. What exactly is the knee protesting about? Well, the condition is well known to runners: it is called *chondromalacia* of the *patella* (kneecap), or "runner's knee".

Chondromalacia is medicalese for the softening of a cartilage in a joint, in this case the kneecap. In young women it is caused by a combination of effects. One theory holds that as the female body develops, the hips spread. The tendons and other soft tissue around the knee do not grow quickly enough to keep up with overall body growth, so a tightness develops, particularly in the *patellar tendon*. As the pelvic area spreads, the thigh bones take a different angle relative to the lower limbs. At the same time, a new awareness of footwear fashion leads to the wearing of all the wrong shoes. And, if the young woman has an over-pronation syndrome, the likelihood of chondromalacia increases even more. The second theory holds that the tendons are actually loose and lax, and therefore the patella is pulled to the outside of the knee when it is fully bent. I believe that both theories are true, as I have seen very convincing arguments on both sides.

The overall result of these effects is that the patella is not properly grooved in the knee joint, and the all-important *Q-angle* is out of kilter (see Diagram 12:11). The knee is being pulled to the inside, and the entire leg is rotating internally, basically on account of the spreading of the pubescent hips and the slow tendon and other soft-tissue development. Dr. Hamilton Hall, the eminent orthopedic surgeon, calls the end result, descriptively enough, the "teenaged female knee-pain syndrome".

In most cases the treatment for this annoying condition is patience, accompanied by specific muscle-strengthening exercises to take the pressure off the knee joint. Orthotics may be required to correct over-pronation and to properly align the foot with the knee. It is also necessary for teenage girls with the condition to wear the proper footwear—preferably running-shoes, and definitely not high heels.

It is only in rare cases, when conservative treatment and time fail to eliminate debilitating pain, that surgery to repair the cartilage damage will be required. I would certainly recommend seeking a

DIAGRAM 12:11
The "Q"-Angle

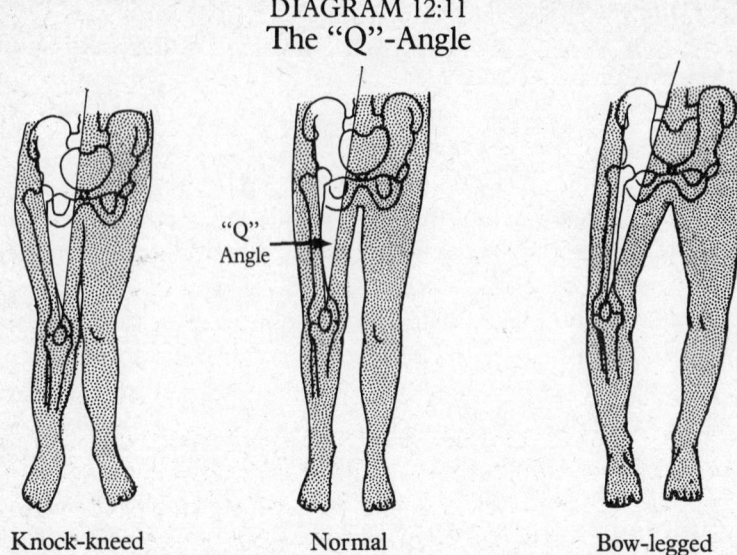

"Q"
Angle

Knock-kneed   Normal   Bow-legged

second opinion if surgery is advised for a young woman's chondromalacia condition before other measures have been taken. With the right exercise program and proper footwear, a teenage female with chondromalacia of the patella ought to outgrow the disorder by the time she finishes high school.

I know that I have not discussed foot problems of adolescents in any great detail. The reason is that most disorders will have been picked up and dealt with before a child reaches grade five. Also, once a child enters the teen-age years, the problems become more similar to those of adults—except for the cases of aseptic necrosis of the growth plate of a bone—and have been discussed in detail in other chapters. The important thing to remember is that children cannot, or will not, always tell you when their feet hurt, so parents will have to be very observant of the way their offspring walk and run. And, if a problem does arise, parents must have it taken care of quickly so that the child does not suffer later on, and is not required to undergo more aggressive treatments. Lastly, I repeat, do not be frightened when an offspring is born with, or develops, an abnormality of the lower limbs. If the condition is caught early, non-surgical treatment is usually the norm, not the exception, and the child will not be exposed to lengthy periods of uncomfortable, debilitating convalescence.

13

For Want of a Shoe That Fits

Roman historians have chronicled that Julius Caesar was determined to make his foot soldiers travel farther and faster, and he reckoned that a change in footwear might improve the speed and agility of his fighting men. One of the things he experimented with was the heel height of their boots. Caesar's best scientific minds eventually discovered that the soldiers marched faster and lasted longer on their feet without tiring when their heels were about one inch high. Caesar's experiments may have been the first logical scientific studies to determine the most comfortable shoe a person ought to wear, but they were certainly not the last. Analysis of the average person's gait has convinced running-shoe manufacturers that the Roman scientists were basically correct—the one-inch heel is the optimum heel-height for a pair of shoes for the average person. If only shoe manufacturers today would pay attention to the facts! Although the wearing of improper shoes may not be the primary cause of foot miseries in modern societies, it can certainly aggravate an existing condition, and cause a few of its own.

One of the problems with footwear selection is that there are some salespeople selling shoes for men, women, and children who know absolutely nothing about feet or biomechanics. They know only about styles.

Would you have a suit or a dress fitted by someone who knew nothing about tailoring? If not, then why would you allow a person who knows nothing about feet to fit you with a pair of shoes? I always tell my patients who are wearing ill-fitting shoes to make sure that the salesperson fitting them knows something about feet. If that salesperson cannot answer questions satisfactorily for them

197

regarding the correct size and shape for them, or about inherent biomechanical problems in certain styles, they are advised to seek another salesperson, or another boutique.

The Shoemaker

Up until the Industrial Revolution shoes were made by a local shoemaker who tailored his footwear to fit the feet of his customers. All shoemakers had their own designs and types of footwear—boots, shoes, etc.—that were their trademarks, but what most of them had in common was their ability to provide comfort for their customers. But now, in industrialized countries, footwear is mass-produced to fit the average foot, not the individual foot. Moreover, the major concern of shoe manufacturers is, logically, turning a profit. Today, shoes are sold on the basis of fashion design, because it would seem that modern man/woman is far less interested in comfort than in style. In fact, I would estimate that about ninety per cent of the North American population will opt for style over comfort when it comes to shoe selection. This sad fact may be good for my business, but it is also frustrating for me because, although I can make my patients' feet feel better, I am unable to keep them that way when they refuse to wear proper shoes. Actually, I am being a bit unfair, because many people would wear shoes that fit them properly if only they could find them.

Approximately eighty per cent of North American males will wear a size-8 to a size-12 shoe of medium width. The same percentage of females will have size-6 to size-9 feet, also of a medium width. Therefore, shoe manufacturers will gear their productions to that eighty per cent of the market to maximize sales and reduce production costs. Many of them will also leave out half-sizes to cut their costs. So, if your foot is not of average size, you may have great difficulty finding the proper shoe for your foot in the size you need and at a price you can afford. As a result, you may settle for a shoe that does not quite fit you properly.

There are shoe manufacturers that do make all sizes and widths, but they generally offer fewer and less-stylish models, because they are usually much smaller enterprises without a large design component. Moreover, even when their shoes are considered fashionable, their output is so small relative to the demand that very few shoppers can find them.

Men are slightly better off than women, perhaps because the styling of men's shoes does not vary much from year to year. That may be due to the fact that heel height is not a major factor in the design of men's shoes, so there is less that can be done to change the style. Also, older men seem to prefer the brogue, or wing-tip, style of shoe. The reason may lie in the fact that—as one of my first male patients told me years ago—brogues most resemble the footwear they had to wear in the armed forces, and they like them because they give them the best support. Whatever the reason for the popularity of certain men's shoe styles, the fact is that manufacturers can produce more shoes in odd sizes knowing that they will eventually be sold— if not this month or this year, then next month or next year. Concurrently, shoe retailers will not panic when the shoes do not sell immediately, because they know the merchandise will eventually be bought.

Women with uncommon shoe sizes are not as lucky as men, because fashion plays a much greater role in the manufacture of women's footwear. This year's style may not reappear again for years, so why should a manufacturer produce extra amounts of odd sizes, and why should shoe retailers stock them when they might be stuck forever with unwanted inventory?

A large percentage of the twenty per cent of women with uncommonly sized feet have the same problem: a narrow heel and a broad forefoot. In order to manufacture a shoe to fit that kind of foot, the producer must make a *combination-last* shoe. "Last" refers to the shape of the shoe. It can be compared to the frame of an automobile. There are two basic types of lasts, *straight* and *curved*, and that fact is important, particularly if you have a foot problem (see Chapter Fifteen). The two things to remember here are that the last should basically conform to the shape of your foot, and that most shoes are single-lasted. A combination-last shoe requires greater production time and costs, and is not as easy to make stylish as a single-lasted shoe.

A woman with a narrow heel and a broad forefoot may have, for example, a heel width that is AA, and a forefoot width of B. Shoes with an AA heel and B forefoot are not easy to find, and when they do reach the stores, as I have mentioned, they are gobbled up quickly by the smart early-bird shopper. Therefore, until shoe manufacturers begin mass-producing a stylish product with a combination last, women who want to wear what they consider to be fashionable shoes that fit them comfortably will have to either shop with an eagle eye or settle for a poorer fit. Unfortunately, too many women in this position opt for style over comfort, and eventually they pay the price in foot problems.

Another factor to consider when purchasing a new pair of shoes is the sizing of particular manufacturers. Every shoe manufacturer uses a different last, just as every car-maker has a different body frame. And, like automobile manufacturers, shoe producers also make many different models. So, for example, the same shoe producer can make a variety of size-9 shoes from totally different lasts. The result is a totally different fit for each model.

Therefore, if a person tells me that he or she is a "perfect" size-8½ fit, I say nonsense, because there is no perfectly consistent size-8½ shoe. One manufacturer's size 8½ is another's size 8 or 9. Keep this in mind when you are shopping for new footwear, and do not hesitate to go up or down a half-size if your normal fit suddenly seems abnormal. In all probability your foot has not changed dimensions, but you are most likely trying on a different-model shoe, possibly from a company whose shoes you have never tried before.

Shoe manufacturers and consumers seem to have forgotten—or choose to ignore the fact—that the primary functions of a shoe are to cover and to protect the foot. (The makers of athletic shoes tend to be exceptions. I will discuss such footwear in detail in Chapter Fifteen.) Actually, if we lived in temperate climates and spent all our waking hours strolling along the beach or walking on soft grass, we would not even require any footwear. We tend to forget that our ancestors never covered their feet; neither do certain tribespeople today.

I wish I could persuade my patients to opt for comfort over style, but I realize that societal norms and values would have to change dramatically before this would happen. And I do not expect shoe manufacturers to altruistically begin mass-producing shoes to fit the foot that is not an average size. So I can only advise my patients to take the extra step and seek out shoes that truly fit their feet well. And I remind them that by choosing fashion over logic, they may well be setting themselves up for future lower-back, hip, knee, and foot troubles that will require much more in the way of medical attention, and cause a lot more discomfort, than the social discomfort of not being fashionable.

What Shoes To Buy

When you shop for a new pair of shoes, remember that price has no relationship to comfort, unless you are seeking modern running-shoes or very soft leather shoes that allow your foot added flexibility.

When you are buying shoes, there are three things that you must take into consideration—besides size. The first is flexibility: Does the shoe allow your foot to bend where it is supposed to bend? The second is stability: Does the shoe keep the foot properly positioned during the gait cycle to lessen the possibility of a biomechanical fault? The third is: Does the shoe provide sufficient shock-absorption to take undue stress off the foot during the stance phase of the gait cycle?

The one type of shoe that comes closest to meeting all three criteria is the running-shoe, particularly the modern one, which has been able to combine flexibility, stability, and shock-absorption without sacrificing too much of any quality. This is one type of shoe that gets better as the price increases, although running-shoes are not nearly as expensive as high-fashion shoes.

I understand why it is that most people are not able to wear running shoes all the time, although it is not uncommon for business people and fashion models to wear them to work, and then switch into fashionable footwear. However, if you have a lower-back, hip, or knee problem, you ought to consider wearing running-shoes whenever you can. They help compensate for biomechanical faults and provide much better cushioning than most other shoes. If you cannot wear running-shoes most of the time, keep in mind that rubber or crêpe soles provide better shock-absorption than other types of soles.

Children's Shoes

Bad habits begin in childhood, often as a result of parental misguidance. There are two problems that come to the fore, and contribute to children wearing the wrong shoes at the wrong time in their development. The first is that old ideas die hard, and children are often forced into shoes that their parents had to wear when they were the same age. I am speaking of those inflexible oxfords that parents used to think were essential for arch support. The second problem is that children become fashion-conscious at too early an age; they want uncomfortable shoes that look pretty or are stylish because they are "in" footwear.

There is no proof that any shoe *except* a well-constructed running-shoe is good for a child with normal feet. And even most children with foot abnormalities are better off with running-shoes and orthotics than heavy, unyielding shoes. If corrective shoes are required, they must be prescribed by a specialist. Do not allow yourself to be talked into any type of shoe inserts for your child by a shoe salesperson. As I mentioned in the last chapter, a child's foot may be harmed by correcting a fault that does not require immediate attention. If you are at all concerned about your child's feet and footwear, have that child examined by a specialist, not by a shoe salesperson who may unwittingly recommend an unnecessary, and potentially harmful, shoe insert.

As far as adolescents are concerned, they tend to wear running-shoes most of the time because they are the most comfortable. However, young girls can develop a bad habit of wearing three-inch and higher high-heeled shoes before they have finished growing, and that can cause problems, particularly with their knees (see Chapter Twelve). Although I am against high-heeled shoes in general, I believe they are particularly harmful to young girls.

Adult Shoes
I have commented throughout this book on the evils of *high-heeled* shoes, particularly those over three inches. The human body was not designed to walk on three-inch or four-inch heels that produce severe anatomical distortions and can result in orthopedic problems from the lower back down to the feet. Back specialists agree that high-heeled shoes are one major cause of backaches in women. High-heeled shoes put abnormal stress on the back of the leg, the knees, and the lower back, and result in shortened Achilles tendons if worn regularly. They also put tremendous stress on the forefoot, which is also probably being squeezed by a tight toe-box. There is little I can add to what I have already said about the perils of high heels, except to appeal again to women to avoid them if possible.

Some heels are even higher than just high. I am referring to those with "*spike*" heels that are at least four inches high and have *sharply pointed toe-boxes*. The only nice thing I can say about these shoes is that they are good for podiatric business. They do everything bad for the foot that three- or four-inch high-heeled shoes with pointed toe-boxes do, only much worse.

Slingback shoes have a strap in the rear to hold the foot in place, and are generally no more than two inches in heel height. Although they provide good breathability for the foot in warm weather, they have no stability in the heel and provide little shock-absorption for the foot. However, they are reasonably flexible and comfortable, and much less damaging for the average foot than high-heeled or negative-heel shoes. An advantage of a slingback shoe is that the heel width can be adjusted by the strap.

The *negative-heel* shoe became popular during the "hippie" years, and was advertised as being "natural". But there was nothing natural about the lower-back and leg pains that they caused. Negative-heel shoes force the Achilles tendon to overstretch, which in turn causes muscles and tendons all the way up into the lower back to overextend. They also produce an abnormal stance phase of the gait cycle, because they force the heel of the foot to remain on the ground too long. This leads to all sorts of biomechanical foot faults. Fortunately, the negative-heel shoe is basically history.

Wooden shoes, or *clogs*, are very popular in certain societies because they provide decent metatarsal and longitudinal-arch support, although they are inflexible and do not provide much shock-absorption. The shoe itself mimics an arch-support, and if you over-pronate it will provide some stability.

My co-writer tried out a pair of clogs, because they were recommended to him by a Dutch friend who said they were good for people with back problems. He wore them twice, and each time he twisted an ankle when he took a bad step and the shoe did not "give" at all. He now sticks to good running-shoes most of the time.

Sandals are very popular in warm climates because they allow the feet to breathe comfortably and therefore remain reasonably dry and cool. However, very few sandals provide much stability or shock-absorption; therefore, they are not recommended for people with lower-limb problems.

High boots are quite fashionable in the winter. It is difficult to rate them as a group, because heel heights vary considerably. The rule of thumb is, then, that they should be treated as high-heeled shoes if the heels are above two inches. The only other thing to mention about such boots is their lack of breathability. Unless they are lined, they are not going to keep your feet that warm, but they will reduce circulation of air around the lower extremities. Therefore, your feet and lower legs may actually feel a bit clammy.

As I mentioned earlier, *men's footwear* is not normally as hard on the feet as are women's shoes. The main concerns in men's shoes are the proper fit, an adequate amount of room in the toe-box, decent shock-absorption, stability, flexibility, and lacing that does not pinch the nerves on the top, front part of the foot. Very few men have heels on their shoes that are higher than one inch. If they do wear high-heeled shoes, they will have problems similar to those of women who wear high-heeled shoes regularly.

The Geriatric Shoe
Finally, older people often have more trouble with their feet than their juniors. Therefore, it is important for them to wear the proper footwear. And, because they often have circulatory problems in their feet, they have to try and keep their feet warm in cold weather to prevent frostbite or immersion foot (chilblain).

It is imperative for such people to find shoe salespeople who know how to fit shoes and offer advice on what stockings to wear in different climates. My advice to them would be to wear good running-shoes as often as possible, because they provide the best overall protection and comfort, particularly when they take walks to exercise. There is no reason why a healthy older person should not be able to enjoy a daily constitutional in comfort, without any footwear concerns.

One final piece of advice I want to give readers has to do with trying on shoes, no matter what the style. I have often heard from patients that they have to break in their shoes, that their shoes are never comfortable when they buy them, but gradually give until they fit the feet. The problem with this theory is that, if they do not fit at first, what damage are they doing to your feet during that time? And why do so many people who argue that their shoes have to be broken in have foot problems? If a shoe does not feel good on your foot when you first try it on, don't buy it! That shoe is obviously not right for your foot—and it most likely never will be. Conversely, if a pair of shoes feels fine at first, but then becomes uncomfortable, don't continue to wear it. You may not feel that you got your money's worth, but you have to accept the fact that the shoes are not right for your feet, and chalk up the purchase to experience.

14
Athletes' Feet

Sports Medicine: A High-Growth, High-Tech Industry

Back in the days before fitness became an international craze, sports medicine was confined to the treatment of injuries suffered by professional or other highly competitive athletes. Those injuries were most often treated by orthopedic surgeons, because bones and joints were the parts of the body thought to be most often damaged by contact, and other demanding, sports. If a weekend or non-competitive athlete had a sports-related injury, the usual remedy was a visit to the family doctor, who might prescribe rest, Aspirin, and the elimination of strenuous activity for all time. How those times have changed!

It is estimated that today in North America there are fewer than ten thousand athletes who might be considered professionals, whereas there are at least seventy-five million people who exercise regularly in one form or another. Therefore, a need has developed to broaden the field of sports medicine to treat these amateur athletes—who are, of course, just as prone to injury as are professionals.

Many of us associate the recent fitness craze with running or jogging (running slowly). In fact, in 1984 a major North American running-shoe manufacturer grossed just under $1 billion from the sale of its shoes. And this company is just one of many in the industry. So you can imagine just how many runners there are out there regularly braving the elements, including midwinter blizzards.

But there are two other types of activity that are very popular these days, and have helped make sports medicine a very lucrative

206

and interesting field. The first of these is the group of racquet sports: tennis, squash, racquetball, and badminton. The second is aerobics, and similar types of exercises. I would estimate that at the S. C. Cooper Family Sports Medicine Clinic at the Mount Sinai Hospital in Toronto, the majority of our patients are runners, racquet-sports players, and aerobic-exercisers. The breakdown would be roughly sixty per cent runners, twenty-five per cent aerobic-exercisers, ten per cent racquet-sports players, and five per cent from all other sports activities. (I will discuss many of these other activities—specifically baseball, skiing, hockey, gymnastics, football, basketball, soccer, and ballet-dancing—later in this chapter.)

There are different reasons for the popularity of these various activities, not the least of which is the desire of the younger generations to get and stay fit. However, racquet sports and aerobics classes are often combined with social activities, and games like squash or tennis satisfy the needs of competitive personalities. But running is a different matter; runners are often totally disinterested in the après-activity scene. They derive their enjoyment from communing with nature, and from what is often called a "runner's high", which is thought to be a result of the body's production of *endorphins*—a person's own opiate. The more you exercise, the more you apparently produce these endorphins; the more endorphins you produce, the less you feel pain and other discomforts, and the more you feel a sense of euphoria.

What does all this have to do with feet? Simply that those of us who run, play racquet sports, or do aerobics often have a tendency to exercise through a pain-tolerance level, and when we do that we are often setting ourselves up for a sports-related injury, because, when something hurts, it is nature's way of telling us that something is amiss and that we ought to stop and rest. Also, we ought to find out what is causing the discomfort. When a person finally gets the message that a part of his or her body is not functioning normally during some form of exercise, we at the Sports Medicine Clinic enter the picture. We now have an average of eighteen thousand patient visits per year at the clinic, and the figure is rising dramatically.

The most common complaint at the Clinic is that of knee pain. Approximately thirty per cent of the patients we see have some sort of knee problem. Right behind the knee is the foot, also near thirty per cent, followed by shin splints and other lower-leg problems at about twenty per cent. About ten per cent of the complaints involve the hip and lower back; an equal percentage involve the neck, shoulders, and elbows.

As you might have already guessed, a large percentage of knee problems and shin splints are directly traceable to poor biomechanics of the lower limbs. The same can also be said for hip and lower-back complaints. This makes me a very busy man at the clinic, and it is gratifying for me to watch the improvement in patients with these disorders as a result of our excellent physiotherapy programs and our ability to correct the biomechanical faults of the feet with the use of the proper inserts.

Many of the lower-limb problems afflicting athletes have already been discussed in detail in this book. Therefore, what I will concentrate on in this chapter is how an athlete acquires the disorder, and how he or she can be properly treated. Serious athletes have to be treated differently from the general population, because their life-styles and psyches demand that they be able to get on with their athletic endeavors as quickly as possible.

Conditions that regularly affect serious athletes, but less commonly the general public, such as shin splints, will be described fully in this chapter.

I would guess that the majority of readers interested in this chapter will want to turn directly to the physical activity in which they are engaged. To that end, I have divided the chapter into categories of physical activities. However, I would advise you to read about all the athletic activities discussed here. Some day you may no longer be able to carry on with your favorite sport, or you may be considering an exercise program for the first time.

Runner's Low

I have rarely seen a sight as forlorn as a dedicated runner derailed by an injury. And what a wide variety of ailments there are to plague a runner—from the toenails all the way up to the spinal column. In fact, the miseries are so numerous, I thought it best to break them down to the parts of the lower limbs and spine that they can affect.

The Black Badge of Courage

Athletes who run long distances, either at one time or over a period of days, can eventually wind up with blackened toenails, in which the color comes from blood that has dried and clotted under the nail. What happens is that the longer a person runs, the more his or her feet will swell from the heat inside the shoe. Therefore, the running-shoe becomes too small after a while and, with each step, collides with the front part of the foot—and the toenails.

As a result of this friction, there is damage to the nail and the nail bed. The nail itself is rubbed by the shoe, and in turn rubs against the nail bed itself. Blisters form to protect the area, and some pinpoint bleeding occurs from the irritation. The blisters may break, and as the fluid from them and from the clotting blood dries, skin around the area will stick to the nail. The end result is damage to the *nail matrix* (the nail-growing cells), which causes the nails to grow abnormally (*gryphotic*). So, a runner with the badge of courage has a blackened, disfigured nail that may never return to normal if damage to the nail matrix is severe.

Obviously, the badge of courage can be at least partially avoided. You can simply stop running long distances, or you can take the preventive step of wearing the best-fitting shoes possible at all times when running, although that is not always a simple matter under certain conditions during lengthy runs. Having an extra, and larger, pair of shoes handy during a long run would be one solution, albeit not a practical one. Perhaps some genius will invent a pair of running-shoes that automatically expand to fit the constantly swelling foot.

A possible side effect of the badge of courage is the development of a fungal infection, since the conditions exist for its growth. Therefore, if you do develop the condition, it would be wise to apply an anti-fungal preparation regularly for the duration of the disorder.

If the badge of courage is allowed to develop untreated, the nail may become so badly damaged that it will fall off. That in itself is not a big deal, and the nail will eventually grow back, although its shape may be abnormal. The positive aspects of the badge of courage are that the disorder is more esthetically unpleasant than dysfunctional and uncomfortable, and it is hardly serious enough to prevent a runner from putting in his or her daily quota of miles, or kilometers.

A Blistering Pace

Athletes are regularly plagued by blisters that form on parts of their bodies which are subjected to undue friction. As an example, I have seen many baseball pitchers in my years as podiatric consultant to the Toronto Blue Jays who have been forced to leave a game because they had developed painful blisters on their fingers from gripping the ball extremely hard in order to throw certain pitches, particularly on hot, humid days.

Blisters are nature's way of trying to protect the inner layer of skin (*dermis*) from becoming inflamed. A watery sac develops in the lining between the dermis and the outer layer of skin (*epidermis*) to prevent inflammatory friction from attacking the inner layer. However, as anyone who has suffered from them will know, the blisters themselves are very sore, particularly if the irritation continues in the area.

Runners develop blisters, and not just under their toenails. The most common areas for blisters on the runner's foot are under the first metatarsal head, and on the ends of the toes. These are areas where the foot is most often subjected to friction caused by over-exercising and by wearing poor footwear.

Blisters are obviously easy to diagnose, and relatively simple to treat, since the cause of the friction that produced them need only be removed. In most cases, all that is required is a change of footwear. Properly fitting shoes and stockings or socks that allow the foot to breathe normally ought to prevent most blisters from forming. If, however, the blisters persist, it may be advisable to try a cheap insole to support the arch and prevent the foot from sliding forward. Another technique to prevent blisters is the use of a product called *Second Skin*, which can be purchased at all sporting-goods stores. First a moisturizing agent, such as petroleum jelly, is applied to the affected area for a cushioning effect to remove the friction. Then the Second Skin is applied over the moisturizer and held in place by medical tape. This product often works well in cases of recurring blisters.

If a person continues to run on blistered feet, he or she will eventually form a callus at the affected areas to protect the dermis. This is another example of nature at work. Of course, the victim will then have another problem to deal with, although the blisters will not normally reappear where they flourished before the callus developed.

One problem that could arise with a blister is the possibility of infection if it breaks. At that point it may become necessary to treat the area with an antiseptic, and to cover it with some sort of bandage. A painful blister may also be deliberately broken with a sterile instrument to relieve pressure. If this is done, however, care must be taken to prevent the development of an infection.

Fore-lorn

Runners are constantly stressing the front part of their feet, and are therefore very susceptible to forefoot injuries. You will recall that in Chapter Six I noted that the forefoot is the workhorse of the foot, because it is in contact with the ground seventy-five per cent of the time during the stance phase of the gait cycle. It stands to reason, then, that runners, who land harder when striding than walkers, are subjecting their forefoot to even more pounding than is the average person.

Because the forefoot is subjected to such pressure, it is not uncommon for a runner to develop injuries such as: metatarsal-head stress fractures, particularly after long runs; neuromas and other nerve-entrapment conditions; capsulitis/synovitis of the metatarsophalangeal joints; and sesamoiditis or fractured sesamoids. And now a new disease has popped up in our high-tech era to plague athletes—the *turf toe*. However, since it rarely affects runners unless they always run on artificial turf, we will save our discussion of the turf toe for later in this chapter.

As I mentioned in Chapter Six, metatarsal stress-fractures occur in runners who have subjected their feet to undue stress, like running too far for too long in the wrong shoes. A runner may hear a "pop" during the run, but will not feel any pain or notice any swelling in the area of the metatarsal head until a few hours later. Then the pain becomes quite noticeable.

I have already discussed the symptoms and treatment of metatarsal stress-fractures in Chapter Six, but there are a few points to make here so that runners will not prolong their discomfort. Metatarsal stress-fractures will heal by themselves under normal circumstances. Abnormal conditions would include trying to run through the injury. The normal recovery time for the fracture is four to six weeks, although it may take older people up to six months to heal completely. But, if you run before the fracture has healed, not only will recovery time be longer, the pain will linger and be more severe. Also, there is a distinct possibility that when the bone does eventually heal, there will be an abnormality left that could eventually cause trouble. So, do not try to be a hero. If you fracture a metatarsal bone, bite the bullet and quit running until the healing process has been completed. A medical expert will advise you when to begin to run again, and suggest other activities that you can undertake in the meantime to keep in decent condition.

Talking Horse-Sense: Sesamoid Problems

Although fractured sesamoid bones have landed many a horse in the glue factory, the same fate hardly applies to humans. However, as you also learned in Chapter Six, a fractured sesamoid can be fairly troublesome, and may have to be removed surgically. If surgery is required, it can be done on an out-patient basis, and the runner should be able to begin running again in about three to five weeks. The same recovery time is usually indicated for a sesamoid bone that has fractured but does not need to be excised surgically. The important thing for a runner to remember, again, is not to try and run through the injury. Also, the runner must be patient, for the sesamoid bone will rarely heal completely. But do not despair; it is not uncommon for a person with a fractured sesamoid to be relatively symptom-free after the inflammation of the break has calmed down. The bone merely remains *bipartite* (in two pieces), but causes no further problems—in most cases. In fact, I have seen only one sesamoid fracture that healed completely in all my years of examining feet. And yet it is the exception rather than the rule to have to remove the fractured bone surgically.

I discussed chronic sesamoiditis in Chapter Six. It is often more difficult to diagnose the inflammation than the break, and just as difficult to treat it aggressively because of the constant pounding even normal walking inflicts on an area that is already inflamed. However, the chronic discomfort and swelling can be reduced by the application of ultrasound, ice, and, if deemed advisable by a medical professional, two cortisone injections given two weeks apart. However, the success rate with all of these treatments is at best fifty per cent. If the inflammation is acute, the injections or non-steroidal anti-inflammatory drugs taken orally may help. If the problem persists, orthotic devices designed to take weight off the forefoot could be of some value. More than likely the inflammation will take its time healing, and the runner will have to be patient for a few weeks and do other exercises that do not stress the forefoot, until the discomfort has disappeared. Women will also have to refrain from wearing high-heeled shoes that put extra pressure on the forefoot.

Nerve-racking
Neuromas, and other nerve entrapments on top of the foot, are not uncommon in runners. Unlike the non-athlete, serious runners will develop neuromas traumatically, rather than gradually over a period of time. Since the pain is in the general area of the metatarsal head, it is often mistaken for capsulitis or synovitis of the metatarso-phalangeal joint (see Chapter Six). However, the latter conditions are more often caused by sports activities other than running. If you recall our discussion of these conditions in Chapter Six, you will know, however, that inflammation of the joint can result in impingement on the nerve running through the affected space between the toes. Therefore, it is possible to suffer from a neuroma and synovitis/capsulitis at the same time.

One of the major causes of forefoot neuromas in runners is running on uneven surfaces for a fairly long period of time, and on a continuous basis. For example, if you run five miles a day for a week on a banked surface, you will be putting terrible excess stress on the meta-tarsal heads, because you are creating an artificial over-pronation situation in one foot. In Toronto, the majority of roads are banked somewhat to allow for water run-off so that the streets will not flood. If a person runs on the inside part of the road, the foot closest to the curb will be a few degrees lower than the other foot. The artificially induced pronation that results puts extra pressure on the metatarsal heads of the lower foot. If a runner already has a slight over-pronation problem, running on city streets could well increase the risk of a lower-limb injury.

This severe pressure on the metatarsal heads can cause a pinching of the nerves in the forefoot, particularly in the areas between the metatarsal bones near the metatarsal heads. This could result in the development of a neuroma. The obvious way to reduce such a risk would be to run on as level a surface as possible at all times.

Another potential cause of a forefoot neuroma is running-shoes that are too tight, either to begin with or after a person has run for a long time and his or her feet have swelled considerably. Obviously, tight running-shoes will force the metatarsal bones to scrunch together and impinge on the nerves passing through the spaces between the bones. The best way to avoid this problem is to ensure that your running-shoes fit as perfectly as possible, and are not tied too tightly. And if you do have a problem with forefoot neuromas, it would be wise for you to stop your running when your running-shoes start to feel uncomfortably tight.

If a neuroma persists despite a change of running conditions and running-shoes, you can try temporary *padding-and-taping* of the offending area to separate the metatarsal bones (see Chapter Six). You should also consider orthotic inserts as a long-term preventive measure to control troublesome neuromas. If the inflammation at the onset of the neuroma is acute, anti-inflammatory drugs or the injection of cortisone (if injected *outside* the joint) may be effective. Surgery to remove the impingement is strictly a last resort.

Calluses, Corns, and Hammer Toes

Runners get calluses, corns, and hammer toes for the same reason as non-runners: faulty biomechanics of the feet and lower limbs. Calluses may also develop on the bottom of the foot—particularly under the toes—in response to the need to protect sensitive areas from friction that causes blisters.

The treatment for these conditions is the same for runners as for the general population. The biomechanical fault must be corrected. For runners, that may involve a simple change of running-shoes, since so many of the modern shoes have built-in supportive devices. However, orthotic devices may also be necessary to correct a biomechanical fault. There is certainly no need for a runner to have to give up his or her favorite pastime just because a callus, corn, or hammer-toe problem persists and has become uncomfortable. With the proper footwear, there is no reason why these conditions cannot be controlled and eventually eliminated. Obviously, there may be cases where a hammer toe might have to be surgically repaired. But, assuming the operation is done properly, a person ought to be able to resume a running program within a matter of weeks.

Midfoot Crises
I have devoted scant space in this book to the midfoot. This is because, as I have mentioned, very little ever goes wrong with its component parts. However, runners and other athletes can injure the area, particularly the tendons that are attached to the midfoot bones (see Diagram 14:1).

DIAGRAM 14:1
Tendons Attached to Midfoot Bones

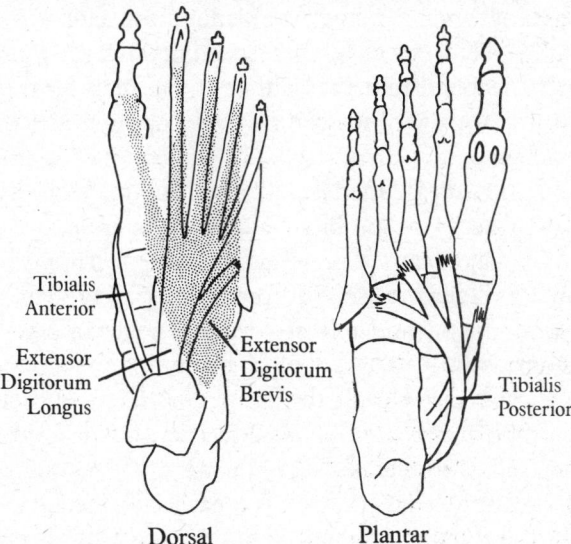

Tibialis
Anterior

Extensor
Digitorum
Longus

Extensor
Digitorum
Brevis

Tibialis
Posterior

Dorsal   Plantar

Tendonitis (inflammation of the tendons) occurs in runners with biomechanical faults that create an imbalance in weight distribution on the foot, and cause muscles to overstretch. As you learned in earlier chapters, muscles are attached to bones by tendons, and these overstretched tendons pull away, or are torn away, from the bones to which they are attached. The tearing, or fraying, of the tendons sets up an area of inflammation that can be quite painful and may require a lengthy healing period.

The four major anti-pronation muscles of the foot are the *tibialis posterior* and *tibialis anterior*, and the *extensor digitorum longus* and *extensor hallucis longus*. When a person is not running, a 3-degree pronation will pose no problem for these muscles. However, runners automatically place extra stress on their feet when they are in full flight, and even a 3-degree pronation becomes excessive and forces these four muscles to stretch to their limits. As a result, the tendons at the ends of these muscles become prone to fraying or tearing. This situation sets up an inflammation at the spot where the tendons are attached to the bones of the feet.

Tendon *sheaths* (the covering of the tendon) generally have a poor supply of blood. Therefore, inflamed and torn tendons do not normally heal quickly. As a result, it is not uncommon for a person who has been running, and has developed tendonitis in a foot, to be advised by the family doctor to give up the activity for all time to allow the tendon to heal and remain healthy. If you have been given such advice, you would do well to seek a second opinion, from an expert in sports medicine.

Because tendonitis is often so difficult to treat, and takes such a long time to heal, the problem ought to be nipped in the bud. Although the major causes of tendonitis in the runner are faulty biomechanics and an overuse syndrome (doing too much, too soon), it can be brought on and exacerbated by neglecting to warm up and stretch properly—if at all—before beginning to run.

Of course, you may do all the proper exercises and still have a tendonitis problem, because of a biomechanical fault in your foot that did not cause problems when you were not running seriously. Therefore, it is important that, at the earliest indication of pain in the foot while you are running, you stop and seek expert advice, particularly from a medical professional specializing in sports medicine.

Once tendonitis has been diagnosed, and the cause has been determined to be biomechanical, the obvious next step is to place an orthotic device in the running-shoe to eliminate the fault—which is usually abnormal pronation. If the tendonitis is acute, you will have to stop running until the inflammation clears up. Anti-inflammatory drugs, ice, and/or ultrasound treatments may help. Once the tendon has healed sufficiently, it would be wise to undertake a proper stretching program to ensure that the muscles and tendons of the foot are in the best possible condition to prevent further trouble. I suggest that you learn these exercises from a sports-medicine therapist.

The tendons of other muscles in the foot are also susceptible to inflammation as a result of irritation caused by a runner's foot that is out of synch. The muscles involved in the midfoot area are the *extensor hallucis longus* and *brevis*, the *flexor hallucis longus* and *brevis*, and the *flexor digitorum longus* and *brevis*. These six muscles can be identified in Chapter Two. They, too, are inflamed either by a biomechanical fault or by an external factor, such as poorly fitting running-shoes or running on uneven surfaces. As with other causes of tendonitis, inflammation of the tendons of these six muscles can be identified by pain in the area of the disorder. Unfortunately, inflammation of these tendons is also equally difficult to treat, unless the root cause of the problem is isolated and dealt with. Prevention is obviously the best medicine.

Pincer Movement

There are three major superficial nerves that run down the top part of the foot: the *medial dorsal cutaneous*, the *intermediate dorsal cutaneous*, and the *lateral dorsal cutaneous* (see Diagram 14:2). These nerves can be entrapped by external factors, such as running-shoes that either are too tight or are laced too tightly. The impingement occurs because the medial and intermediate dorsal nerves, in particular, are very close to the skin and are exposed to trouble as a runner's foot expands during a long run and is rubbed by the tight shoe.

The symptoms of these nerve impingements are pain in the immediate area of the pinching, numbness, and a pins-and-needles sensation both at the site of the entrapment and also into the tops of certain toes. If the medial nerve is involved, there may be numbness and tingling in the first and second toes; with impingement of the intermediate nerve, in the second, third, and fourth toes; and with the lateral nerve, in the fourth and fifth toes. Entrapment of the dorsal nerves is easy to distinguish from entrapment of the nerves

DIAGRAM 14:2
Cutaneous Nerves of the Dorsal

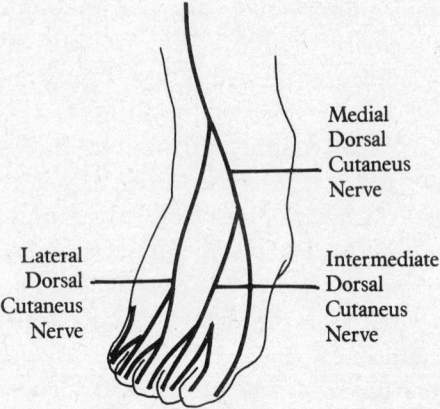

running between the toes (neuromas), because the pain, numbness, and tingling sensations are all felt on top of the foot and the toes, not beneath them.

Because entrapment of the dorsal nerves is almost exclusively caused by tight running-shoes, the obvious treatment is to wear better-fitting footwear—and not to lace them too tightly.

Heel Hath No Fury . . .

About twenty-five per cent of all the patients I see at the Sports Medicine Clinic have heel problems—either plantar fasciitis or Achilles tendonitis. I have already discussed both disorders in detail, but it may be appropriate to remind you that the Achilles tendon is attached to the heel bone at the rear of the foot (see Diagram 8:3). It is when this tendon is inflamed at the heel bone that tendonitis develops. In runners this condition is far more prevalent, because, as mentioned, a person can pronate up to three degrees while walking, without any side effects, but a runner will begin to experience difficulties with the degree of pronation because the foot is being subjected to greater stress than the walking foot. Also, runners have a tendency to overuse and/or under-prepare themselves when they run. I suggest that you perform a proper set of exercises for the Achilles tendon (actually for the calf muscles that lead down into the tendon) before running.

I discussed plantar fasciitis in detail in Chapter Eight. You will recall that the plantar fascia is a soft-tissue mass connected at the front part of the heel bone and at the metatarsal bones (see Diagram 8:4).

Plantar fasciitis is caused primarily by abnormal pronation. However, improperly fitting running-shoes, running on uneven rather than level surfaces, or doing too much running up and/or down hills can also cause mild pronation problems. Occasionally a mild pronation problem can be produced or aggravated by the constant switching of running-shoes. The old adage "If the shoe fits, wear it" applies to running-shoes. Constantly changing your running-shoes will result in constant changes in weight-bearing patterns on the foot, a situation that could cause biomechanical problems. I have seen a few patients at the Sports Medicine Clinic who changed shoes as often as they changed socks, and who developed biomechanical problems because of the regular switching. The time to change a running-shoe is when it no longer feels comfortable, or when you have developed a definite foot disorder, not merely when you feel like a change for no particular reason.

I discussed the symptoms of both Achilles tendonitis and plantar fasciitis in Chapter Eight, as well as the treatment for both conditions. The added advice I have for runners is not to run through pain in the back of the foot, and to seek the help of sports-medicine experts when you think that you have either problem. A good sports-medicine doctor, with the help of a therapist trained in sports medicine, will be able to get you back on track with a sound treatment and rehabilitation program.

I can recall the first severe case of Achilles tendonitis I saw at the Clinic four years ago. The man had a thirty-month history of pain and failed physiotherapy treatment behind him and this had left him convinced that the only alternative was surgery to try and repair the tendon. He had actually scheduled elective surgery, but came to the Clinic on the advice of a friend. When I saw him literally walking on his ankles while in his running-shoes, I was convinced he had a severe biomechanical fault. We prescribed custom-made orthotics for him, and, to make a long story short, he never required surgery. The Achilles tendonitis eventually disappeared on its own. This man's experience led us to examine all patients with Achilles tendonitis for biomechanical foot faults, and our clinical experience to date, based on over three hundred cases, indicates that approximately eighty-five per cent of all cases of chronic Achilles tendonitis may respond favorably to orthotics. This is why I believe that runners, and other athletes, with heel problems would probably be far better off if they took their complaints to a sports-medicine clinic, or to any expert in sports-related injuries of the lower limbs.

Of course, there will always be cases of Achilles tendonitis that are not caused by biomechanical faults, or that are caused by them but do not respond to orthotic treatment. This leads me to argue strongly that the best way of handling the disorder is to prevent it from happening in the first place.

Preventive measures are not that difficult to follow. The runner must wear proper footwear. Women who have worn high-heeled shoes all their lives, and then begin a running program, will have to take special precautions, because the high heels have caused their Achilles tendons to shorten. So they will have to stretch their tendons properly before they begin running. Actually, it is an excellent idea, as I have already mentioned, for all runners to properly warm up and stretch their Achilles tendons before they begin running. It is also important at the end of the run to stretch the muscles again after they have "warmed down" to prevent them from over-contracting.

Out of Joint

Although ankle troubles are more common in sports other than running, a runner can sprain the joint, often severely, by taking a bad step. It could happen on a surface that is not level or on one that is fairly rough, particularly when you are running at night and cannot always see the danger.

A sprained ankle is actually a sprained ligament. Ligaments have very little give, although they are reasonably flexible, so they cannot naturally lengthen to accommodate pressure placed upon them. If you were to "turn" your ankle as you were running, you would place undue stress on the ligaments of the ankle joint—remember that a ligament is a fibrous band of connective tissue that links bones together at a joint. When this happens, the ligament is either stretched beyond its limits and becomes "sprained", or else, in the worst scenario, it is torn completely away from its moorings (see Diagram 14:3). When the injury first occurs, it is often very difficult to properly diagnose as a tear or a sprain, because the swelling and the pain in the area prevent proper manipulation of the joint. The only way to adequately manipulate the area would be to put the patient under a general anesthetic and then play with the ankle. However, such a procedure is rarely, if ever, necessary.

DIAGRAM 14:3
A Severe Inversion Sprain

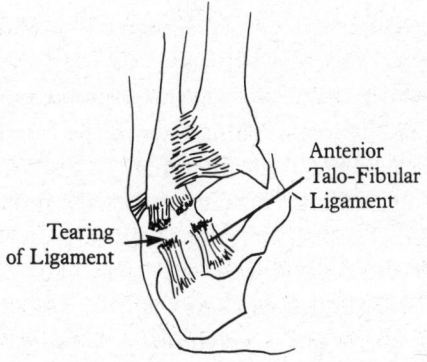

There are three ligaments in the ankle area that are commonly stretched or torn when the ankle is "turned" (inversion sprain). Two are shown in Diagram 14:3. The one most likely to be damaged is the *anterior talo-fibular ligament*.

Incidentally, I get a lot of questions concerning the ankles from people who are running indoors, or on small outdoor tracks or paths. If you are constantly turning on a track that has, for example, a dozen or more laps to the mile, are you more prone to overstressing the ankle than if you run on a long, straight pathway or a quarter-mile track? The answer is a qualified yes.

Indoor tracks, in particular, are often well banked at the corners to conserve energy and cut times for the runners. While you may run farther faster, the problem with these tracks is that the banking produces excess pronation in that leg and foot that are higher on the turn than the other leg and foot. So, the possibility exists of exacerbating a biomechanical fault that already exists, or even creating one. Such a fault, like over-pronation, will eventually result in increased pull in the muscles, tendons, and ligaments in the ankle area—and in other parts of the leg and foot.

If you do run indoors, try to avoid severely banked tracks. Also, alternate directions frequently so as to avoid stressing one leg too much. This may cause traffic jams on the track, but that is better than sore ankles or knees. Of course, if you change directions repeatedly, but still run for a long time on a steeply banked, very hard surface, you may wind up with damage to both lower limbs.

The general philosophy for the treatment of a sprained ankle can best be summed up by the acronym "RICE". In this case it does not stand for a dish in an Oriental restaurant. *Rest*, *Ice*, *Compression*, and *Elevation* are the four main components of the treatment, at least for the first three days after the injury. Rest is necessary to give the ankle area a chance to calm down; any weight on the offending foot will only exacerbate the inflammation. Ice is essential to keep down the level of swelling caused by the inflammation, and it also acts as an analgesic to reduce the level of pain. Compression, or the bandaging of the injured area, aids in keeping down the swelling and the internal bleeding caused by the injury. Elevation of the foot allows for improved venous and lymphatic flow out of the area. This reduces swelling in the area, and therefore limits the loss of motion in the ankle joint.

There is a special way to tape the ankle when one of its ligaments has been damaged. The artistry is known as a *high basket weave*. This method of bandaging the area provides excellent support for the ankle joint, and enables the injured person to put weight on the foot again much sooner than if a conventional tensor bandage were to be applied. This type of bandage should be left on for about a month, although it must be removed and re-applied periodically to allow the area to be examined, and to let the skin "breathe".

Providing that the proper treatment was begun at the outset of the injury, physiotherapy can be started two to three weeks after the accident, even in cases of moderate to severe ankle-ligament sprains. Ultrasound works well, and should coincide with stretching exercises to allow the ankle joint to return to full mobility as soon as possible. And, most importantly, special exercises are required to return to normal the *proprioceptors* of the ankle. Proprioceptors are sensory nerve-endings that monitor the internal changes in the body resulting from movement, particular muscular activity. When the ankle joint is injured, the proprioceptors in the area are damaged, and the ankle appears to have been weakened, because the offending foot continues to be unstable. I wish I had a hundred dollars for every time I have seen patients who have been told that their injured ankles were not healing properly, because the ligament had not returned to normal. In most cases the ligament has healed properly, but the proprioceptors are still unable to inform the foot where the rest of the leg intends to go. As a result, the foot does not land where it is supposed to when a person is walking, and the results can be painful and/or comical, depending on whether you are the victim or the spectator.

Synovitis of the Ankle Joint
As you know from Chapter Six, *synovitis* is an inflammation of the outer lining of a joint. Sometimes abnormal pronation can cause the head of the tibia to impinge on the ankle joint, particularly in the case of runners who can exaggerate a biomechanical fault when they constantly pound their foot on hard pavement when running. The result can be ankle-joint synovitis. Ice, ultrasound, and other forms of therapy will not do much good in the long run, because the biomechanical fault must be corrected in order to eliminate the cause of the inflammation. Therefore, the best way to obtain permanent relief from the synovitis caused by a biomechanical fault is to be fitted with a proper shoe insert.

The Tarsal-Tunnel Syndrome
We discussed this ailment in detail in Chapter Eight—particularly how difficult it could be to diagnose. The condition involves the impingement of the *posterior tibial nerve* in the area of the *deltoid ligament* on the *medial* (inside) side of the foot (see Diagram 8:8). A runner can develop numbness and tingling sensations in the area of the pinched nerve, and along the bottom of the foot and the toes, because abnormal pronation strains the ligament, which then begins to press on the nerve. However, it takes about three to four miles of running before the symptoms appear, and for that reason

it is most difficult to diagnose, unless the runner with the problem jogs directly into the doctor's office after a lengthy, painful run.

As I mentioned in Chapter Eight, the primary treatment for the tarsal-tunnel syndrome is the wearing of correctly fitting running-shoes and orthotic devices. In rare cases, the nerve may become so inflamed by constant impingement that surgery may be required to widen the tarsal tunnel and/or redirect the nerve through a less congested area.

Because running is so unforgiving of abnormal pronation—the non-runner can often get away without symptoms with up to a five-degree pronation, whereas a runner will suffer the consequences of even a three-degree pronation—I rarely see tarsal-tunnel syndrome in non-athletes. And, fortunately, I see only five or six runners per year with the syndrome.

Taking It on the Shin

Shin splints have become one of the bread-and-butter items for sports-medicine clinics, particularly with the present popularity of aerobics. (I will have more to say about aerobics later in this chapter.) Although this disorder has been in the medical spotlight for the last few years, very few people actually know what it is, and how it is caused.

Shin splints are known in medicalese as *periostitis*, because it is the *periosteum*—the dense outer layer of connective tissue that covers bones, except where they articulate—that is damaged when it is pulled away from the bone by a tendon to which it is attached.

Although shin splints occur well above the foot, they may be caused primarily by our old friend abnormal pronation, compounded by repeated landings on hard surfaces, which place tremendous shock-absorbing stress on the lower extremities.

There are two types of shin splints. The first, and most common, type is called *anterior tibial shin splints*; the second is *lateral tibial shin splints*. As you can see in Diagram 14:4, the first type of shin splints is caused by an abnormal pulling force of the *tibialis posterior muscle* where it is attached to the *tibia* (the shinbone). The second type of shin splints is caused by the *tibialis anterior muscle* where its tendon attaches to the tibia.

The tibialis posterior muscle works in the leg to prevent abnormal pronation. It can become overworked when a person who is over-

DIAGRAM 14:4
Anterior and Posterior Sites of Splints

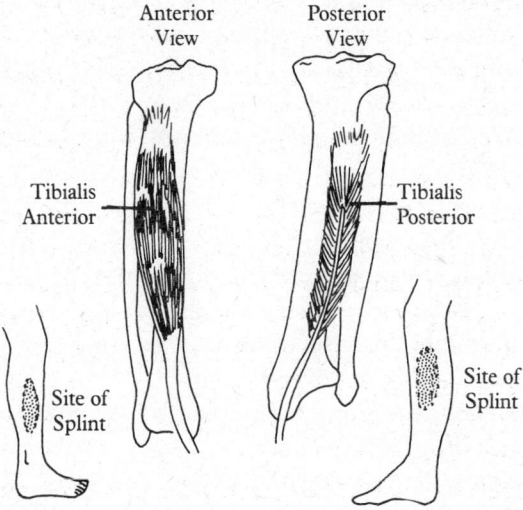

Anterior
View

Posterior
View

Tibialis
Anterior

Tibialis
Posterior

Site of
Splint

Site of
Splint

pronating is engaged in strenuous activity, such as jumping up and down, or running for long periods. Eventually the muscle and its tendon are pulled so tight that the periosteum of the bone becomes stressed, and may tear away from the bone, producing the condition known as shin splints. This inflammation makes the affected area of the tibia extremely tender, and the discomfort can last for up to six months in severe cases, until the periosteum reattaches itself to the bone.

The tibialis anterior muscle is also an anti-pronation muscle, but it is affected more by abnormal forefoot pronation. Shin splints caused by the stress on this muscle and its tendon can be distinguished from posterior tibial shin splints by the site of the inflammation (see Diagram 14:4).

There is one other cause of shin splints aside from abnormal pronation. I have seen many people who, through disuse, developed chronically shortened muscles and tendons in their legs over a period of years. Then they suddenly decided to jump into some form of athletic endeavor without preparing their bodies for the rigors of the exercise. As a result, their muscles and tendons were forced to overstretch to cope with the activity. When this happens to the tibialis posterior and tibialis anterior muscles, shin splints are likely to develop.

Treatment for shin splints will then depend partially on the cause of the condition. If abnormal pronation is to blame, correction of the biomechanical fault is essential, along with physiotherapy to relieve the inflammation. If the problem is one of a new athlete doing too much too soon, the soft tissues of the body will have to be prepared to withstand the stresses of strenuous exercise. Also, it is important for a runner to run on level surfaces that are not too hard, to reduce the risk of over-pronation, and to reduce shock-absorption stresses. Running-shoes have to have the proper support to prevent the foot from "rolling" too much when it lands. Finally, running uphill is bad for shin splints because it places extra pressure on the toes, and can exacerbate forefoot over-pronation.

If a person has succumbed to shin splints, ice and ultrasound will help relieve the inflammation, and proper stretching exercises are a must to prevent a recurrence of the problem. If shin splints are ignored, and allowed to worsen, they can cause a micro-fracture of the tibia or the fibula. We see about fifty cases of these stress fractures at our Sports Medicine Clinic every year. Therefore, I strongly advise you not to try to exercise through shin splints. If you do, you will only set yourself up for bigger troubles.

The Anterior-Compartment Syndrome

If you are not an athlete or a medical professional, you may never have heard of this condition. The *anterior-compartment syndrome* can be confused with shin splints because, as you can see in Diagram 14:5, the anterior compartment (medicalese for "a part or section in the front") is in the front part of the lower leg.

An acute anterior-compartment syndrome has, in the past, been considered as a medical emergency, because no blood reaches the compartment owing to a pinching off of the major artery providing oxygenated blood to the area. But, since the advent of sports medicine as a discipline of its own, anterior-compartment syndrome has come to mean many different things. Now any pain in the area, such as an anterior tibial shin splint, is often diagnosed as an anterior-compartment problem. As you can see by Diagram 14:5, there are many muscles in the anterior compartment with different smaller

DIAGRAM 14:5
The Anterior Compartment

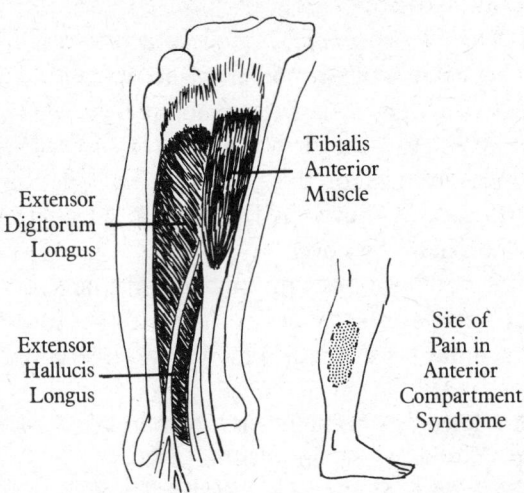

Extensor
Digitorum
Longus

Tibialis
Anterior
Muscle

Extensor
Hallucis
Longus

Site of
Pain in
Anterior
Compartment
Syndrome

compartments between them. When any of those muscles inflame and swell, they increase the pressure within these compartments. This increased pressure may cause a mild decrease of blood-flow and, therefore, some mild pain. This is what occurs ninety-nine per cent of the time, and it is rare for surgical intervention to be necessary.

If the condition is mild, the discomfort and inflammation can be alleviated with rest, ice, and easy stretching of the leg. But it can recur, unless the cause of the problem is addressed. The most common causes are poor biomechanics of the lower limbs; ill-fitting shoes; ineffective or insufficient warm-up, stretching, and cool-down exercises; and overuse (doing too much). I would advise all runners, and, indeed, all serious athletes, to pay attention to the need for proper exercising before and after you engage in strenuous activity in order to avoid a potential anterior-compartment-syndrome problem, particularly if you have a biomechanical disorder.

If the anterior-compartment syndrome persists, despite all the treatment and preventive measures, it may be necessary in the most serious chronic cases to operate to *decompress* the compartment— to enlarge the space through which the impinged blood vessel must pass. However, this would be a rare occurrence, so there is no need for you to worry unduly if you suffer from the syndrome but have not yet taken all the steps necessary to control it.

The Chondromalacia Generation

When I first began practicing podiatry and sports medicine in the mid 1970s, there was very little written about *chondromalacia patella*, alias runner's knee. And the first time I ever heard about the "Q-Angle" (the measurement of the *patellar tendon* in relation to the leg and the kneecap, as shown in Diagram 12:11), I thought I was being told about a new spy novel.

However, the popularity of running/jogging, and other stressful activities like aerobics, has resulted in a rapid increase in this syndrome, which has in turn led to increased research into its causes and treatments.

The runner's-knee syndrome has its roots in the abnormal motion of the kneecap. As you can see in Diagram 14:6, the kneecap normally sits comfortably within the groove that lies between the *medial* and the *lateral femoral condyles* (rounded protuberances at the ends of some bones). The back of the kneecap is covered with cartilage that normally glides smoothly in the groove, but if the kneecap were to move off-center in that groove during its motions while a person is in stride, it would rub against the sides of the groove, much like a bowling ball racing erratically down the gutter of the alley.

When the kneecap no longer moves within normal limits in the groove, the cartilage begins to rub against the surfaces of the condyles (also Diagram 14:6). The result is wear-and-tear on the cartilage. If it is allowed to progress, the bone beneath the cartilage will eventually come into direct contact with the bony condyles. The resulting friction will lead to a gradual breaking down of the joint.

Although runner's knee will not necessarily show up on X-rays, particularly early ones, there are some obvious symptoms of the condition. The irritated area becomes swollen and inflamed, and acute pain radiates from the top of the kneecap. Stiffness can occur when a person has been sitting with a bent leg for over two hours, and the pain will become quite pronounced when a person is going up or down stairs. In severe cases, there will be occasional *painful* grinding in the joint when the knee is bent. (However, *painless* cracking within the knee joint itself, or for that matter in any other joint in the

DIAGRAM 14:6
Kneecap Positions

Front View (Normal)

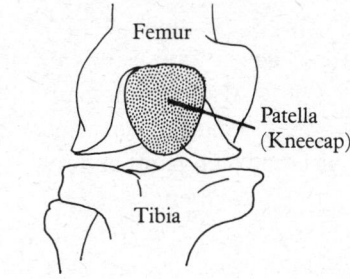

Femur

Patella
(Kneecap)

Tibia

Skyline View

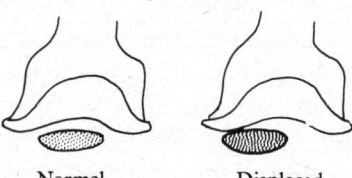

Normal   Displaced

body, is, as far as most orthopedists are concerned, of no significance, and is certainly not symptomatic of any knee disorder). Finally, there will be a general loss of patellar mobility as a result of the chondromalacia. In other words, your knee will just not do all the things you want it to do without difficulty and/or pain.

There are three major causes of runner's knee, assuming the joint and the kneecap themselves are normal, and sometimes they all act together to promote the condition. The three are: weak or malfunctioning *quadricep muscles* above the knee, faulty biomechanics of the foot and lower leg, and a dysfunctional *patellar* tendon below the knee. I will concentrate on the biomechanical problems.

A foot that abnormally pronates tends to turn a person's knee to the inside. When that happens, there is undue stress on the knee joint itself, and the kneecap may deviate from its normal path in its groove as the leg tries to compensate for the abnormal pronation.

Another factor in the development of runner's knee may be the poor alignment of the patellar tendon with the knee joint. One of the reasons may be abnormal pronation, which forces the tendon out of alignment as it attempts to compensate for the biomechanical fault.

There are a few less-common causes of runner's knee. A person may be running in ill-fitting shoes that by themselves induce a biomechanical fault. Or the runner may be running on banked, uneven, rough surfaces that can accentuate a biomechanical fault and cause pulling on the knee joint. Also, running up or down hills will add to the stress on the knee, which is constantly bent to adjust to the sloping terrain. It has been determined scientifically that the forces on the leg multiply threefold when a person runs uphill, and fivefold when running downhill. So it is easy to understand why runners, and other serious athletes, are far more prone to foot and leg problems than non-exercisers.

When I see a case of runner's knee, the first thing I must do after making the diagnosis is to find the cause. This is done by taking a complete case history, examining how the patient is walking, determining the anatomical structures of the lower limbs, and discussing the patient's training and exercise habits. Once I have determined the cause of the complaint, I can then advise the patient as to the proper corrective measures and therapy to take.

If the cause is a biomechanical foot fault, the insertion of orthotics in the running shoes is indicated. Also, it is essential that the runner be advised of the proper shoes to wear. I will discuss athletic shoes in detail in the next chapter.

Many people with runner's knee have found relief with the use of various braces, straps, and other similar paraphernalia to keep the knee joint in proper alignment. These appliances may indeed help relieve mild pain, but they do not correct the underlying causes of the disorder. Therefore, I would strongly recommend that a person seek expert medical advice before relying solely on such aids to treat runner's knee, or any other knee condition.

Tibial Pursuit

Runners who are slightly bow-legged (*tibial varum*) or knock-kneed (*tibial valgum*) will be prone to problems to which they would not be subjected under normal walking conditions. This is, of course, because of the extra stress placed on the legs while running, particularly on hilly or uneven terrains.

One of these problems is osteoarthritis of the knee. Keep in mind that this is a wear-and-tear condition, not a disease. If the runner is bow-legged, all of the body weight may be transferred to the *medial* (inside) *compartment* of the knee, because of an inverted position of the feet to compensate for the shape of the leg. If the problem is one of knock-knees, the runner may over-pronate and force the body weight onto the *lateral* (outside) *compartment* of the knee (see Diagram 14:7). When these conditions occur, the overstressed side of the knee joint wears down while the other side remains as good as new.

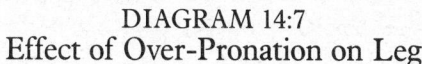

DIAGRAM 14:7
Effect of Over-Pronation on Leg

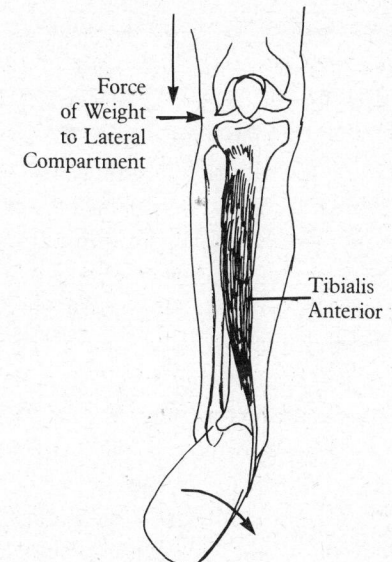

Force
of Weight
to Lateral
Compartment

Tibialis
Anterior

Because wear-and-tear disorders are painful, osteoarthritis in the knee joint will produce discomfort in the area of the inflammation. X-rays of the knee joint should confirm the presence of the condition.

The treatment for this situation is to reduce the inflammation with physiotherapy and/or oral anti-inflammatory drugs. At the same time the biomechanical fault of the lower limbs must be dealt with. Orthotic devices will compensate for over-pronation or abnormal supination, and will help keep the legs as straight as possible. It is important to exercise the quad muscles and the hamstrings, as they also help keep the leg properly aligned. If some permanent wear-and-tear has occurred, modern surgery techniques may be able to repair much of the damage. It is important for athletes to remember that if they are experiencing pain in the knee area during exercising, they should seek medical advice as soon as possible to determine the cause of the problem, and to avoid the potentiality of a lasting disorder in the knee joint.

And the Band Frayed On

The *ilio-tibial band* is a stretch of muscular tissue that runs from the hip joint down the outside of the leg and attaches into the head of the fibula, just below the knee (refer to Diagram 14:8). One function of this band is to prevent internal rotation of the leg and thigh, and it is vital for runners, because they place heavy, repetitive stress on their legs with every stride.

If the ilio-tibial band, which runs over the outside part of the knee joint, is stretched too tightly, it will become irritated by the friction occurring when it contacts the kneecap. The band may be overstretched, because if it is poorly developed or very short, it is abnormally tight to begin with. Also, a badly over-pronating foot will produce an internally rotating leg, and that situation will also stress the band unduly. Occasionally the *ilio-tibial-band friction syndrome* will be caused by too much hill-running, or by running constantly on uneven, rough terrain.

The symptoms of the syndrome are pain and tenderness on the outside of the knee at the head of the fibula, and upwards. The symptoms may approximate runner's knee, because walking up and down stairs produces pain, and there is stiffness in the knee joint after a person has been sitting with knees bent for more than a couple of hours. However, that pain will be more on the outside of the joint. Some medical experts believe that the discomfort is caused by an inflammation of the *bursa*, the small sac of fibrous tissue, filled with synovial fluid, that is situated in areas where there is friction caused by ligaments or tendons that pass over bones. In this case, the bursa lies between the tendon and the lateral side of the knee (also Diagram 14:8).

DIAGRAM 14:8
The Ilio-Tibial Band and a Bursa Site

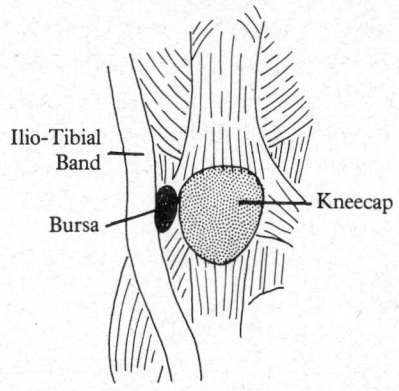

The treatment for ilio-tibial-band friction syndrome is a program of exercises to properly stretch the band, ice and ultrasound to relieve the discomfort, a change in footwear, possibly including the use of orthotics to correct a biomechanical fault, and a change in running habits to avoid more stressful conditions.

A Pain in the Butt

There has been controversy recently in medical circles about the existence of a disorder known as the *piriformis syndrome*. I have no doubt that the condition does exist, since we have treated over three hundred cases of it in the last few years at the Sports Medicine Clinic—with encouraging results.

The *sciatic nerve* exits from the spinal column and runs down the leg. When it is pinched either in the low back or somewhere in its path down the leg, it produces aches, pains, and occasional numb, tingling sensations down the leg and into the toes. The discomfort is called *sciatica*.

Until recently it was thought that all cases of sciatica originated with an impingement of the sciatic nerve in the lower back, caused by a protruding *disc* or *facet-joint breakdown* in the spinal column. But many specialists now believe that the nerve impingement can take place in the upper part of the leg, specifically where the nerve runs under the *piriformis muscle* (see Diagram 14:9). This muscle acts to prevent the femur (thigh bone) from internally rotating, a problem that occurs in runners with biomechanical faults in their lower limbs. When the femur over-rotates, excess stress is placed on the piriformis muscle, which then tightens and binds down on the sciatic nerve. The nerve becomes irritated, and pain from the inflammation radiates from the source of the problem, in the area of the buttocks, and can travel down the leg, behind the knee, and into the foot.

DIAGRAM 14:9
Sciatic Nerve and Piriformis Syndrome

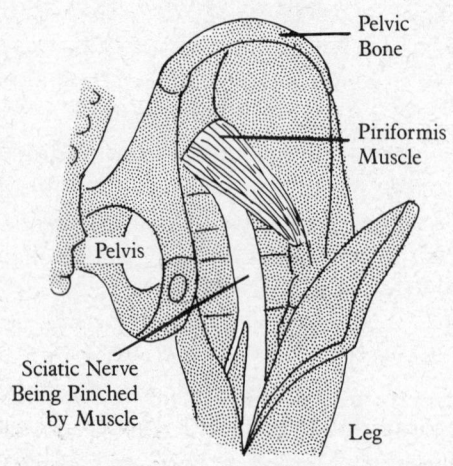

Our clinical experience has been that when we correct the internal rotation of the femur with orthotics, we have had an almost ninety-per-cent success rate in controlling the sciatic pain. Naturally, we take this course of action only after an exhaustive examination of the patient has ruled out a lower-back problem. We also advise the runner to undertake a proper exercise program to stretch the piriformis muscle to prevent it from impinging on the sciatic nerve. A good athletic therapist will provide you with the proper set of exercises.

I suspect that, like runner's knee, we will be hearing a lot more about this syndrome in the next few years as clinical studies are published that lend credence to the theory that the condition actually exists, and is becoming more common as more and more people take up running.

Aerobics: The Twenty-Minute Wear-Down

It is time to turn our attention to *aerobics*. Many condition-conscious people have decided against running as a way of developing their bodies, and have turned to aerobic exercising. I suspect that the reason may be more social than anything else, since aerobics classes are usually conducted at co-ed health clubs where people of both sexes can display their wares and make new friends.

I am inclined to describe aerobics classes as a social disease, because too many unfit people join clubs and immediately jump into these classes totally unprepared for the strain to which the exercises subject their bodies. And, alas, there are too many aerobics teachers on the circuit who do not know how to properly conduct a class, and who are unwilling or ill-prepared to tailor their classes to the needs of their charges.

There are also those people who do aerobic exercises at home to the beat of the instructor on video-tape or television. There are two major problems with this type of exercising. First, there are no instructors to tell you if you are doing something wrong, and are therefore likely to hurt yourself. Secondly, many people try to do too much too soon, in order to keep up with the tapes, or with the unbelievably fit instructors on the television screen.

Please do not get the idea, however, that I am against aerobic exercising. I only caution you to do the exercises correctly, and in accordance with your physical condition. Aerobics are a marvellous way of getting into shape and helping you to shed unwanted weight, without having to go on a starvation diet. Moreover, by increasing your cardiovascular and pulmonary capacities with this vigorous exercising, you stand a good chance of feeling better mentally and physically, and therefore you are better able to cope with the anxieties of life in the fast lane. And, who knows, you may even meet the love of your life in one of these sweaty exercise classes.

The most common concern for those who do aerobics is shin splints because of the tremendous amount of stress to the lower extremities from repeated bouncing up and down during the exercises. A few pages ago, we discussed how the periosteum—the tough outer layer of soft tissue that covers the tibia (the shinbone)—is being torn away from the bone by the abnormal pulling force of the tibialis posterior or tibialis anterior muscle, where its tendon attaches to the tibia. We also discussed how abnormal pronation, in particular, puts extra stress on the involved tendon to try and keep the leg straight during any form of exercising that involves constant pounding on the feet. Well, in aerobic exercises, the feet absorb a tremendous number of repeated shocks. Therefore, the possibility is excellent that shin splints will develop. In fact, recent studies have shown that almost forty per cent of all those who do aerobics at least three times per week will develop shin splints at least once a year. Even more amazing is the fact that almost eighty per cent of all aerobics instructors will succumb to shin splints at least once a year, assuming that they teach at least three classes a week.

Yet people who do aerobics need not develop shin splints on a regular basis. All they have to do is take the proper precautions.

First of all—and I hate to keep harping on the same theme, but it applies to all athletes all of the time—do not try to do too much too soon. Most aerobic injuries are caused by the "overuse" syndrome—overexercising parts of the body that are ill-prepared for the stress. So, if you are a beginner and have joined a club that does not have beginners' classes, but only classes at one level, ask for your money back quickly, and seek out another club that will provide classes tailored to your needs.

It is equally important that, even in beginners' classes, the instructor knows how to properly conduct warm-up and stretching classes so that your body is prepared for the more difficult routines that follow. As far as the lower extremities are concerned, it is vital to stretch the tibialis anterior and posterior muscles and the Achilles tendon before you begin bouncing around the floor. Otherwise you could end up with Achilles tendonitis or a related problem.

Even if you do not have a biomechanical foot problem, it is essential to wear the proper footwear when doing aerobic exercises. Otherwise you will not have the stability to prevent your feet from "rolling" too much, or doing other silly things, during the routines. Remember that biomechanical faults that do not cause trouble when you are merely walking will suddenly cause all sorts of problems once your feet are subjected to additional stresses and are forced to absorb much more shock than normal.

Another common problem for people doing aerobics is Achilles tendonitis, often because the tendon is not properly stretched before the class gets into the difficult routines. And, once again, there is the problem of overuse—doing too much too soon. Women in particular are prone to this complaint because many of them have worn predominantly high-heeled shoes for years, then suddenly have decided to take up aerobic exercising to get their bodies back into shape for whatever reason. As a result, they are trying to do the exercises on Achilles tendons that have shrunk from misuse during their years on the high heels. So they develop inflamed tendons and are forced to give up exercising altogether until the tendonitis clears up, weeks later. By that time they have probably, sadly, given up exercising for good. And all because they did too much, too soon, on Achilles tendons that were not properly stretched before they were subjected to the undue stress of the exercises.

You will recall that stress fractures of the tibia and the fibula can occur when tendons attached to them become so inflamed that they exert tremendous force on the bones. When that force becomes overwhelming, the bone gives, and stress fractures occur. The two major tendons involved with these types of stress fractures are those of the *tibialis posterior* and *tibialis anterior* muscles (see Diagram 14:10). These fractures can take up to a year to heal. One of the problems involved with recovery is mis-diagnosis of the fractures, because they do not always show up on X-rays. Therefore, the patient is often treated first for shin splints, because the pain is in the same area. However, the tell-tale sign of a fracture is the fact that the application of ultrasound to treat the supposed shin splints will enhance the pain, rather than relieve it. It may then be necessary to do a bone scan to isolate the break, although after a few weeks it ought to show up on regular X-rays.

The best treatment for stress fractures of the tibia and the fibula, and for the metatarsals, is prevention. Do not try to exercise through pain; pain is nature's way of telling you that something is amiss in your body. None of these fractures will have to be put in a cast, so esthetically you will not suffer. But the discomfort from the fractures

DIAGRAM 14:10
Two Major Tendons Involved in Stress Fractures

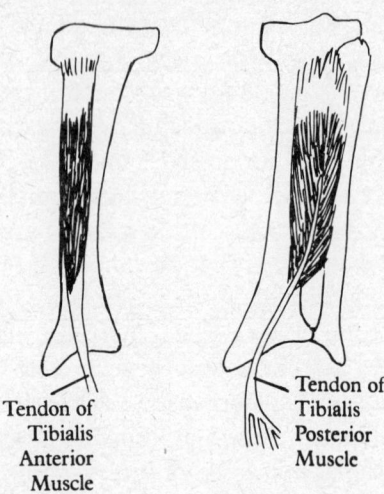

Tendon of
Tibialis
Anterior
Muscle

Tendon of
Tibialis
Posterior
Muscle

can be quite acute and can last for a few months.

Racquet and Ruin

Racquet-sports injuries certainly help pay the bills for any sports-medicine professional, and damage done to the lower limbs of racquet-sports players ranks right up there with those from running and aerobics. The major reasons for racquet-sports injuries to the legs and feet are the dramatic stop-and-start movements required to chase the balls, the hard surfaces on which the games are played, and the lack of proper conditioning of the players. In tennis there is, as well, an increased risk of sesamoiditis because of the great amount of pressure on the first-metatarsal-head area while serving. Professional tennis players, who often serve over a hundred times per match, are quite prone to inflamed sesamoids because these bones lie right under the first metatarsal head. You can imagine just how the biomechanics of the tennis serve stress the area.

Because of all the lateral stop-and-go movements made by racquet-sports players, "inversion" ankle sprains are not uncommon for them. The same lateral movements place an extra work load on the Achilles tendon, which is already working hard to prevent ankle instability, and can cause Achilles tendonitis. The dramatic stopping-and-starting, combined with hard running on unyielding surfaces, can cause plantar fasciitis, because the racquet-sports player is constantly "planting" the heel of the foot for stability and leverage when making a shot.

In the forefoot, racquet-sports players are quite prone to toenail problems, because the sudden stops cause the ends of the toes to slam into the front of the shoe. Aside from the toenails, the bottoms of the forefeet are subjected to tremendous pressure as the player slides laterally from side to side, thereby creating friction between the foot, the shoe, and the court surface. Therefore, it is not uncommon to see competitive players with feet full of calluses and blisters. And, because of the extra stress on the forefoot, racquet-sports players are also more likely than others to suffer from forefoot neuromas. The entire forefoot is being constantly impinged by all of the rapid, jerky movements required in a fast-moving match, and the nerves in the forefoot are fair game for irritation caused by the suddenly cramped spaces through which they must pass.

Finally, the entire lower part of the body of a racquet-sports player is subjected to extra pounding by the constant running and stop-and-start actions on hard surfaces. Therefore, any biomechanical fault that might otherwise not bother a person will probably create havoc in a racquet-sports athlete. I have treated one tennis player continuously for years for various foot and leg problems. He tells me that he can play all day on clay surfaces, because they are yielding, and therefore less demanding in terms of shock-absorption. However, he can play only a few minutes on an asphalt court before he starts to experience all sorts of aches and pains, all the way up to his lower back.

Ballet: To Dance and Pay the Piper
Although ballet dancers may not qualify as athletes, they are certainly as well-conditioned and aware of their bodies as any sports enthusiast. I have treated a number of ballet dancers for various foot problems over the years, and they are definitely in better shape than many of the serious athletes I see in my practice. However, ballet dancers also have foot and leg problems, although these are basically *accumulated* injuries developed during years of continuous straining of

the lower limbs to perform certain movements for which the body was not designed. They also often have muscles that are overdeveloped, because they are required to prevent instability in the feet while dancing.

The most common problem in dancers is hammer toes. Because there is a tremendous amount of pressure on the toes in ballet-dancing, the flexor and extensor muscles of the toes become overdeveloped and tight. When this happens, all the toes contract, and the hammer toes form. Of course, the only way to really prevent this occurrence of hammer toes is to stop dancing on pointed toes. But then what would be left of ballet-dancing?

As you might expect, another common complaint of ballet dancers is osteoarthritis of the toe joints, because of the tremendous stress to the joints during dancing. It is almost inevitable that ballet dancers will suffer early wear-and-tear of the toe joints.

The third major condition affecting ballet dancers is traumatized toenails. If you spent a good part of your work day on your toes, you would also suffer from toenail abnormalities. Ballet dancers are plagued by all three of the most common toenail problems—ingrown, mycotic (fungal), and gryphotic (misshaped) nails. These conditions are the badges of courage for ballet dancers—the price they have to pay for the rewards of their profession.

Ballet dancers also tend to develop soft corns between their toes, because the toes are constantly being squeezed together, and friction in the area between the toes will cause corn growth to protect the irritated skin.

Because ballet dancers are in excellent condition most of the time, and know how to properly warm up and stretch, they usually avoid debilitating injuries, unless they have some sort of accident, like taking a misstep and twisting an ankle, or being dropped or stepped on by a partner. However, they can suffer from various types of tendonitis, strictly from overuse of their lower limbs during exhausting training and/or performances.

Aside from ballet, other types of dancing can be just as hard on the lower extremities. Moreover, other dancers are rarely as fit as ballet dancers, but they often try moves for which their bodies were neither designed nor prepared. Certain forms of modern dance, and acrobatic exercises like breakdancing, are very hard on the lower limbs. So it is not uncommon to see these other dancers with severe cases of plantar fasciitis and shin splints because they have not properly exercised before doing strenuous dances.

Basketball and Volleyball

I have lumped these two sports together because most of the complaints seem to be similar in nature, and are caused by the same types of problems.

Basketball and volleyball players tend to be prone to plantar fasciitis and Achilles tendonitis, because they do not properly stretch their lower limbs before beginning to play. There is a lot of jumping and stop-and-start movement associated with these sports, and the lower limbs will be subjected to a lot of undue stress if the stability of the ankles and feet is undermined by underdeveloped muscles and tendons. Coincidentally, these athletes suffer from sprained ankles as a result of inverted landings after jumping for a ball.

The remedy for these conditions is a proper exercise program to develop the muscles and tendons around the ankle to provide the required stability in the area. If you have had an ankle injury, you would also want to do the exercises I mentioned earlier in this chapter for the *proprioceptors*.

Basketball and volleyball players also tend to be more susceptible to capsulitis under the metatarsal heads than other athletes. This is probably due to the added stress placed on the forefoot as a player prepares to jump for a ball. If a biomechanical fault exists in the forefoot, it will be exaggerated by this preparatory setting of the feet, and it should therefore be treated with a proper shoe insert.

Football

Most of the foot injuries in football are traumatic. Players get stomped on, accidentally or otherwise, or they twist their ankles in unyielding turf. Actually it is amazing, considering the mayhem that occurs during a football game, that there are not more severe, debilitating injuries suffered by the players. One of the reasons may be that football players have exceedingly strong thighs and lower legs. Therefore, their well-developed muscles prevent more than the reported amount of joint and muscle/tendon injuries. Strong muscles help keep joints in their proper alignment; properly stretched muscles help prevent tendonitis.

Football linemen tend to suffer from capsulitis of the metatarsal-head joints because they place tremendous stress on their forefeet when they dig into the turf for leverage to push an opposing lineman out of their way, or when they are trying to stand their ground. It is important for them to treat any existing forefoot biomechanical problem, so that it will not be accentuated by the stresses of the game.

The other problem that football players, and other athletes playing on artificial turf, have to contend with is that of *turf toe*. This is not a dermatological problem; the affected toe does not take on a grassy appearance. It is a condition brought on by the unyielding quality of artificial turf that has been laid down on a field, supposedly to provide better traction and shock-absorption.

Unfortunately, artificial turf has very little give. When an athlete "plants" a foot in order to change direction or obtain leverage, it tends to stay planted. When this happens, the big-toe joint can be jammed and an irritation develops. This irritation of the cartilage in the joint can develop into synovitis or capsulitis, particularly if the athlete repeatedly jams the toe while trying to make a "cut"— to quickly change direction by planting one foot firmly in the turf.

In the good old days of sports fields made of real grass, when an athlete made a "cut" there was enough give in the turf to prevent the toe from jamming when he pushed off the foot. And, if the ground was slippery/wet, he would lose his grip on the turf and slip or fall down. But there would be no undue pressure on the big-toe joint.

Treatment for turf toe is difficult as long as the athlete is playing on artificial turf. However, certain steps can be taken.

First, it has been clinically proved that those athletes most likely to suffer from turf toes have plantar-flexed first metatarsals, the biomechanical fault in which the first metatarsal stays down at all times instead of moving in unison with the other metatarsals during a normal gait. Thus there is more weight on the first metatarsal head than there ought to be, and the area receives greater stress than is normal. This means there is an increased chance of an inflammation occurring, particularly when the area is traumatized. Therefore, it would be prudent for an athlete with such a condition to have it treated with an orthotic device, particularly when he or she is playing a lot on artificial turf.

It would also be wise for a player prone to turf toe to wear shoes with shorter cleats so that they will give way rather than dig deeper into the turf and cause the big toe to jam more.

If the condition requires therapy, ice and ultrasound will often help relieve the inflammation. If the condition is severe, it may be necessary to treat with an anti-inflammatory drug taken orally.

A turf-toe condition, if left untreated, can lead to hallux limitus or hallux rigidus. Once that happens, the player may eventually require surgery to alleviate the discomfort (see Chapter Four).

Gymnastics

Gymnasts are usually in excellent condition, when they are fully mature physically. The problem is that there are too many youngsters in serious gymnastic training who are trying to do too much before their bodies have properly developed. Therefore, they are overstressing muscles and tendons that have not kept up with bone growth. Muscles and tendons that are too short to securely attach to fully developed skeletal forms become overstressed and inflamed. So it is not uncommon to see repeated cases of Achilles tendonitis, plantar fasciitis, and ankle sprains in these youngsters as a result of this overuse of their underdeveloped bodies. Prevention here is worth a few kilos of cure. It is important for still-growing youngsters to get the proper coaching so that they are not being forced to over-extend themselves.

Another problem for gymnasts, young or otherwise, is that of meta-tarsal-head capsulitis. The reason is that there are certain positions on the balance beams, or during floor routines or jumping maneuvers, that place extreme pressure on the forefoot. As with all other strenuous physical activities, the problems of poor biomechanics are exponentially multiplied, compared with normal walking. So it is logical for any gymnast with a foot problem to ascertain whether or not a biomechanical fault exists, and to treat it accordingly at once.

Hockey: If You Want To Skate Like Gretzky

Hockey players are somewhat like football players: they tend to have extremely strong, flexible lower-limb muscles and tendons as a result of strenuous exercising. Therefore, it is not often that I see a hockey player with an injury similar to those incurred by runners and aerobic exercisers.

Most foot injuries to hockey players are traumatic: they get slashed by an "errant" stick or hit by a puck travelling at the speed of sound. Or on rare occasions they may get gashed by another player's skate.

Those players that I see usually have a pronation problem. Although there has been very little research done on the biomechanics of skating, I have noticed that skaters who over-pronate tend to skate with their legs wider apart to compensate for poorer-than-normal balance. Because of this technique, they cannot easily turn quickly or sharply, and their overall ability to compete suffers.

I have seen dramatic improvement in the skating abilities of some hockey players after they have been prescribed orthotic devices for their skates. They may not suddenly become Wayne Gretzskys, but their new-found mobility on ice may save them a few long bus trips to minor-league towns.

Figure skaters are similar to hockey players in that most of the injuries they are likely to suffer will be of a traumatic nature. However, I have treated five world-class figure skaters in Canada who suffered from forefoot neuromas because their skates either were too tight to begin with, or were laced up too tightly. Because their skates were too tight, these skaters placed even greater pressure on their forefeet during spins, and similar moves that place extra stress on the balls of the feet. The obvious solution to the problem is to wear proper-fitting skates and not to lace them up too tightly.

Skiing

You may be surprised to learn that most serious downhill skiers who compete in slalom or downhill events wear orthotics in their ski boots. According to one study I have seen, the figure was about eighty-five per cent, and this cannot be too far from accurate since there are at least a half-dozen major manufacturers of ski equipment that make special orthotic devices for ski boots. These companies would not be producing these products as a tax write-off.

The reason for downhill skiers to wear orthotics is that in a normal run down the slopes they are constantly pronating three or four degrees on one foot while simultaneously supinating the same amount on the other foot. The biomechanics of downhill skiing are such that this phenomenon cannot be avoided. Since a skier would have to have perfectly balanced feet with absolutely no abnormal pronation or supination to be able to tolerate the simultaneous extra pronating and supinating of opposite feet without developing a serious lower-limb problem, it is natural that most of them would require the use of orthotics when skiing. So, if you have a definite biomechanical foot fault, and do a lot of downhill skiing, you would be wise to purchase a pair of special ski-boot orthotics to avoid all the potential overstress conditions that may eventually affect your lower limbs.

There are many ski shops that sell ski-boot orthotics. I have been in many of these stores where the sales personnel knew a lot about the wide range of orthotic devices they carried, and why they were required. But I have also been in a few ski shops where the personnel knew absolutely nothing about the biomechanics of skiing. Therefore, I would make absolutely sure that I was dealing with a ski-equipment store that had well-informed salespeople.

Aside from the biomechanical problems inherent in downhill skiing, forefoot neuromas may develop from ski boots that are too tight. As with any footwear, if the boot does not feel comfortable, get into a size and style of boot that keeps your foot stable, but does not pinch anywhere. I can never understand why some people are so eager to squeeze into the tightest possible pair of shoes or boots they can find. They are only looking for trouble.

Almost all the other downhill skiing injuries are traumatic, the result of attempting too difficult a slope, of using a faulty piece of equipment that causes you to lose your balance, or of just plain bad luck, like running into a tree that refused to get out of your way.

Cross-country skiers rarely have any injuries that can be related directly to overuse or biomechanical problems. This may be because these athletes are like ballet dancers and martial-arts athletes who know how to take good care of their bodies. Also, soft snow is much more forgiving than rigid, hard surfaces, so a misstep is less likely to lead to a disastrous accident that could affect the lower limbs to any great degree.

Soccer: A Fun Game To Boot

Soccer is probably the one truly universal game. Almost every country on earth entered a team in the qualifying rounds leading up to the "World Cup" championships in 1986. And, although it seems to have flopped professionally in North America, it is being played more and more by youngsters as a substitute for the costlier, and more injury-producing, game of American football.

Soccer players can develop an interesting list of foot injuries, aside from the usual plantar fasciitis, ankle sprains, Achilles tendonitis, and similar overuse syndromes. But there are fewer overuse injuries to soccer players than to players of most other sports because they tend to be among the best-conditioned athletes in competitive sports. They have to be able to stand the pace of ninety minutes of constant motion up and down the field. However, they are prone to some injuries, just by the nature of the game, which requires sharp turns, quick stops and starts, kicking the ball from awkward angles, and "tackling" opponents. The condition of the playing surface will often be a factor in a soccer injury to the foot. Rough, hard, uneven surfaces may result in a player taking a misstep, twisting an ankle, and possibly damaging an Achilles tendon or a ligament severely in the process. In North America, many of the games are played on artificial turf, and soccer players are just as susceptible to turf toe as other athletes playing on such surfaces.

Soccer players can suffer from severe tendonitis of the tibialis anterior muscle when the foot is bent awkwardly back from a mis-kick in which the foot accidentally jams into the ground before the ball. Soccer players may also be plagued by lateral shin splints, because they make more use of the outside of their feet, particularly when "dribbling" the ball as they move forward or laterally. They may, as well, develop tendonitis on the *proneus longus* and *brevis* muscles that lie on the outside (lateral) part of the leg. These muscles act to prevent inversion of the ankles, and are strained when a player is kicking the ball sideways. The way to help prevent these inflammations from occurring is to ensure that the muscles and tendons are properly stretched before the game.

Baseball: So Fair and Foul a Game I Have Not Seen
You might have thought that, since I am the consulting podiatrist to the Toronto Blue Jays baseball team, I would dwell on baseball for pages. However, injuries to the lower extremities are not a major concern for most ball players, although a few players have been plagued by, or had their careers ended by, various foot injuries.

One of the most famous, and eccentric, players of all time, Dizzy Dean, was apparently forced to quit after the big toe on one foot was broken by a line drive off the bat of an opposing player to whom he was pitching. He supposedly tried to return to action before the toe healed properly, and altered his pitching biomechanics to avoid the pain in his foot caused by his old, natural delivery. As a result he "threw out" his arm, and his career ended abruptly, long before it should have.

Baseball players today are in much better shape than they were even ten years ago. This is because they now spend much more time warming up and stretching before a game. However, the game has also developed negatively as far as a player's lower limbs are concerned. The culprit is the artificial surface on so many of the stadium floors these days. Major-league ball players now play up to 162 games a year, and often go for days without a break. For those teams that play at home on artificial turf, the toll on the legs of their players is amazing. Because the artificial turf is so unyielding, even the best-conditioned baseball players will eventually succumb to overuse syndromes, such as plantar fasciitis, chondromalacia of the patella, and, to a lesser extent, Achilles tendonitis. I can think of a whole host of major-league players who have suffered a great deal in the last few years from the wear-and-tear on their lower extremities caused by playing repeatedly on unforgiving artificial turf.

Of course, one of the primary scourges of baseball players is the turf toe. They are constantly jamming their big toes into their shoes as they try to change directions sharply and quickly on the artificial turf.

So, while baseball players today are in much better condition than their predecessors of just a few years ago, they are also being battered and bruised more regularly, because of the constant pounding on their lower limbs from running on artificial turf.

Amateur baseball players, and professionals who are lucky enough to play most, if not all, of their games on natural grass, have a very low incidence of foot problems. Because the health of their feet is important to their success as ball players, they tend to take good care of them, and seek relief for nagging hurts that generally turn out to be caused by biomechanical problems. I would suspect that a fair number of baseball players wear orthotics of some kind, but I have never seen a survey to back up my contention.

Traumatic injuries in baseball are usually caused by errant cleats of an opposing player that gash the foot. Unless the cut is deep, it is hardly a serious problem, although the area may be sore for a few days. Some players will twist an ankle sliding into a base, or turn or sprain an ankle while running. Such injuries can take time to heal, but with modern taping techniques and physiotherapy, the player should be back in the line-up within a matter of a few weeks. Some players have a tendency, while batting, to foul pitches off their ankles and shins. Many of them now wear a shin-and-ankle guard when batting to prevent the ball from making a nasty impression on the part of the foot or leg that it hits.

A Pitch for Prevention

When it comes to performing the activity of your choice, there are two things to keep in mind. First, establish your goals—long-term and short-term—so that you accomplish what you have set out to do in a realistic manner. It would be wise to seek expert advice, perhaps from a coach or an instructor, so that you do not bite off more than you can chew. A trainer is also important to help you avoid athletic injuries. Improper training methods are the primary causes of sports injuries, not traumatic episodes. A good coach will be able to provide you with proper warm-up and stretching exercises, and teach you what to do to cool down and keep your muscles and tendons stretched after you have finished for the day. And a coach will refine your techniques, in whatever activity you pursue, so that you will be able to maximize your energy resources while at the same time minimizing the risks of overuse and wear-and-tear syndromes. I have refrained from including specific exercises in this book, because I would rather have an athlete be shown the exercises by an expert—so that they are done properly. If you are unable to obtain the help of an expert, you may get valuable advice from magazines devoted to specific athletic activities, such as running or racquet sports.

Finally, there is an old expression: "Enough is as good as a feast." That expression applies to physical activity, as well as to food. One of the most common causes of sports injuries is the overuse syndrome.

But, if you do injure yourself, by either overuse or trauma, remember that it is not wise to exercise through the pain. You will only aggravate the condition and force yourself out of action for much longer than if you had taken the proper precautions at the onset of the discomfort. Pain tells you something is wrong. It is not to test your character.

15
Athletic Footwear

Athletic-footwear companies are playing a major role in lower-limb injury prevention, not necessarily for altruistic reasons, but because the market is so competitive these days that they have to try and stay a step ahead of the field. As a result, millions of dollars are being spent each year by the industry to produce the perfect shoe to give different athletes ultimate performance. Just as automobile racers rely on certain tires for a competitive edge, so do athletes rely on footwear to give them an advantage over the competition. Also, certain athletic events require different types of shoes, because stresses and ground surfaces differ. And, since every athlete has different feet, one shoe last will suit one runner but not another.

The end result is that there is no longer any such thing as the all-purpose sneaker, except for children who are not playing specific sports.

All this competitiveness and research has led to a much better product for the athlete, but at a much higher price per pair of shoes. However, let me assure you that when it comes to athletic shoes, you do get what you pay for, almost all the time. The major decision for the athletic consumer today is how to choose the proper pair of shoes from among the proliferation of models and manufacturers.

Because athletic shoes today are *sports specific*, you would be well advised to find a store that carries a wide variety of shoes for all sorts of activities and employs sales personnel who are familiar with the merchandise and the needs of specific athletes. If you have a definite biomechanical problem in your lower limbs, you would be wise to consult with a podiatrist who is an expert in sports medicine. Then you will know better exactly what type of shoe to look for. You must also take into consideration the type of surface on which you will be exercising. Different terrains, court surfaces, or playing fields will call for different types of shoes. What you want to avoid is buying the best-looking, highest-priced athletic shoe without taking any of the above into consideration. If you have any doubts at all about the type of shoe you ought to be wearing for a certain activity, keep shopping until you find a knowledgeable salesperson. Remember that although a certain shoe may feel okay when you try it on in the store, it may be totally inadequate for your needs when you are exercising.

There are three major factors to consider when purchasing athletic shoes: *cushioning*, *stability*, and *flexibility*. Recent developments in the designing and manufacturing of such shoes have resulted in footwear that is far superior to that of even ten years ago, and the added stability, flexibility, and shock-absorption have provided more comfort than any other type of shoe made today. So it is not unusual to see business executives, male and female, wearing running-shoes to work. They make the switch to regular shoes only when they reach their offices. We ought, therefore, to take a closer look at a typical modern running-shoe to find out exactly why it helps protect the feet and legs from injury.

Cushioning (Shock-absorption)

Most of the cushioning is absorbed through the midsole that spans the length of the shoe (see Diagram 15:1). The thickness of the highly resilient material that is used for the cushioning generally runs from approximately one inch at the heel to a third of an inch to half an inch at the forefoot. The additional thickness at the heel allows for the extra stress during the "heel strike" phase of the gait cycle. It will reduce the risk of trauma to the heel area, and to the Achilles tendon. Some shoes also have a built-in cushioning system on the outer sole where contact is made with the ground during the running stride. This space-age cushioning has certainly cut down on the number of traumatic overuse injuries to the foot of the runner, particularly in the heel area.

DIAGRAM 15:1
The Anatomy of a Running-Shoe

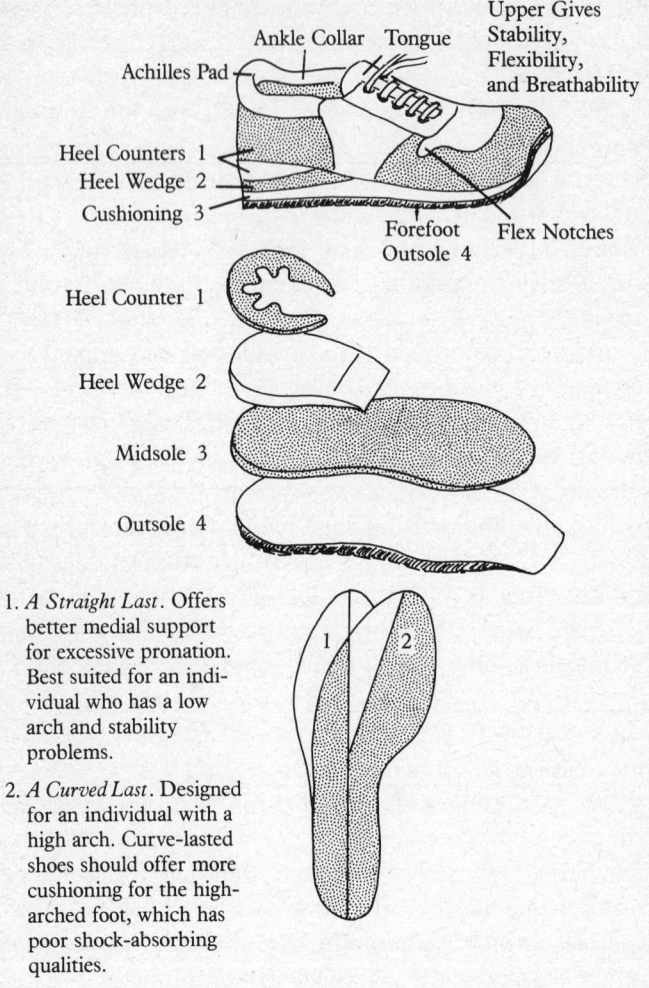

1. *A Straight Last*. Offers better medial support for excessive pronation. Best suited for an individual who has a low arch and stability problems.

2. *A Curved Last*. Designed for an individual with a high arch. Curve-lasted shoes should offer more cushioning for the high-arched foot, which has poor shock-absorbing qualities.

Stability

The modern running-shoe also features high-tech extra-stability devices to improve foot control. The more foot control the shoe offers, the less chance there is of wear-and-tear disorders caused by stressful, repetitive motions. However, running-shoe manufacturers are still unable to provide maximum stability in a shoe without making some sacrifice of cushioning properties, and vice versa. Also, there is often a trade-off of stability for a lighter-weight shoe. Many runners would rather have the comfort of a lighter shoe than have the added stability. If they do not have any foot problems, they can easily get away with this trade-off.

A lot of shoe manufacturers have combined different-density foams in the midsole to provide greater rigidity in various areas. Firm internal and external heel counters (see Diagram 15:1) have also been added in some shoes for more rearfoot control.

One of the most important factors determining stability in a shoe is the *last*. As I mentioned in Chapter Thirteen, the word "last" refers to the shape of the sole, and it can be compared to the frame of an automobile, before the chassis is mounted on it. The two most common types of lasts are *straight* and *curved* (also Diagram 15:1).

There are a few rules that govern the choice of either type of last. First, if the shape of your foot is basically straight, and if you have a low arch, the straight-lasted shoe is best for you, because it offers more support on the inside of the foot, and will help prevent your foot from over-pronating and therefore enable you to minimize pronation-caused injuries.

If your foot is slightly curved, if you have a higher-than-normal arch when standing, and if you have been diagnosed as having a rigid foot, you will probably feel more comfortable in curve-lasted shoes. These shoes offer more cushioning but still retain rearfoot stability. People who over-supinate often find these curve-lasted shoes are much better because the shape of their foot and that of the shoe are compatible.

If you are uncertain as to which type of last to get, you might want to seek expert advice before buying your next pair of athletic shoes. Many runners, though, can tell just by walking in a new pair of shoes for a few minutes whether they require a straight or a curved last.

Flexibility
Flexibility in a running-shoe is necessary to take excessive strain off the muscles in the lower leg while you are running. More flexible shoes provide better shock-absorption, although they may provide less stability.

When shopping for a pair of running-shoes, you should try bending a shoe in half at the midfoot area. If this cannot be done easily, try another pair. You can also determine flexibility by examining the *forefoot outsole patterns* on the bottom of the shoe and looking for *flex notches* on the sides (see Diagram 15:1). These patterns and notches are not there for esthetic purposes; they are designed to provide the shoe with the required flexibility—most importantly in the area of the metatarsal heads and toes.

Other Footwear Factors

There are a few other factors to consider when purchasing a running-shoe, particularly the *breathability* of the shoe, especially in the upper, forefoot part. You do not want too much moisture to be trapped inside your shoe; fungi and blisters thrive in hot, moist areas.

You will also want to know what sort of traction the outer sole provides. You do not want to be slipping and sliding when you are running.

Is the shoe you are choosing light in weight, but still able to provide you with the stability you need? Generally speaking, the lighter the shoe, the less stability it has to offer.

Is there cushioning around the ankle that includes the Achilles pad (see Diagram 15:1) to prevent irritation to this area and consequent skin eruption? Is the tongue of the shoe padded to prevent the laces from pressing on the top of the foot?

Finally, is there a removable inner sole in case you must add your own special orthotic device?

Racquet Sports and Aerobics Shoes

Many of the remarks I have made above refer specifically to running-shoes, which are designed to support a foot that is constantly moving *forward*. They are not designed for repeated bouncing up and down on one's toes, or for quick lateral movements. Therefore, sports activities that require a lot of lateral movements necessitate a shoe that provides more lateral support for the foot. Also, many activities, such as aerobics exercises, place additional cushioning stresses on the forefoot, so they require shoes with additional shock-absorption qualities in the front.

Racquet sports involve repeated, quick, stop-and-go movements in all directions. Running-shoes do not provide for such movements, particularly because of their added cushioning in the heels, and the lack of lateral stability in the forefoot. Raised heels make the back part of the foot less stable. Therefore, quick lateral movements can result in sprained ankles. So, if you wish to minimize the risk of a lower-limb injury while playing racquet sports, buy shoes specifically designed for such activities. There is no place on the court for a running-shoe.

There are many problems that make foot and leg injuries the constant companions of aerobics exercisers. The exercises are usually done on a fairly hard surface. Exercisers spend a lot of time on their toes and, depending on the instructor's routines, moving laterally. Lateral movement is particularly accentuated when aerobics is combined with dancing in *dancercises*. So, an aerobics exerciser must have an exercise shoe that combines added forefoot cushioning with flexibility and stability. Aerobics-shoe manufacturers are continuing their research to develop the perfect product, and for people who are not prone to leg and foot problems, and who exercise on surfaces that have some resilience, the modern aerobic shoe is fine. But for those of you who are constantly plagued by problems such as shin splints, or who are forced to exercise on hard, unyielding surfaces, I recommend that you stick to good running-shoes at this time, because you require the cushioning that even the best aerobic shoe cannot yet offer. I would definitely avoid wearing a racquet-sports shoe for aerobics, because they are made for lateral mobility and fail to provide the adequate flexibility and shock-absorption required for aerobic exercising.

Other Sports Footwear

The major manufacturers of athletic shoes are now branching out. Not only do they make running, aerobics, and racquet-sports shoes, but they produce footwear for every imaginable athletic activity. It would not be feasible in this book to discuss in detail every type of sports shoe on the market today. I can only advise an athlete to consult with his or her trainer/coach, or a knowledgeable sports-shoe salesperson, and to try on the few models available for specific sports, in order to determine the best possible shoe to buy. The rule should be, if the shoes do not feel comfortable during the physical activity, do not wear them at all. The lower limbs can be injured, and overall performance will suffer if the shoes do not fit comfortably.

Finally, some athletes worry about whether they should buy all-leather shoes, or shoes that are half leather and half nylon mesh. All-leather shoes are more durable, obviously, but they are also heavier. The half-and-half shoes are lighter and provide greater breathability for the foot. You must weigh the trade-offs for yourself, and buy the shoes with which you feel the most comfortable. There is no noticeable difference in performance between the two types.

The Asphalt Jungle
Humans may be the only animals that do most of their running and walking on hard, man-made surfaces like concrete and asphalt. Of course, I am referring to modern man, particularly those who live and work in urban areas, and rely on roads and sidewalks for level surfaces on which to exercise or get back and forth. This is a shame, because grass or a level dirt path would provide far more shock-absorption than pavement. But where can one find a nice level path of grass or dirt on which to run in the city?

It is imperative that the surface on which you run be free of pot-holes or sudden, sharp dips, and not overly canted. One bad step on an uneven surface could result in a severe ankle or knee-joint injury. In most urban areas, such a grassy or dirt terrain is difficult or impossible to find. Therefore, runners train on sidewalks or roadways. However, they often neglect to take into serious consideration the pounding to which their bodies are being subjected as they run on hard surfaces. The most important thing they ought to do is wear running-shoes that provide the best shock-absorption qualities.

Extra shock-absorbing material in running-shoes will reduce considerably the jarring forces to which the body is subjected with each stride. It is the added shock of a hard landing on the foot that accentuates biomechanical foot faults, and can lead to injuries such as stress fractures.

The floor on which aerobic exercises are often done is another surface that has been blamed by sports-medicine specialists for the development of problems caused by excessive shock to the foot and leg. The major injury involved here is shin splints. Fortunately, fitness clubs have begun to recognize the problem, and have sought more resilient surfaces to install in their exercise areas. They have found that not only will their members remain more injury-free, but their instructors will miss fewer classes because of shin splints. As I mentioned above, if you are doing aerobic exercises on a very hard floor, you should wear running-shoes, because they provide the best shock-absorption for your feet.

16

Question Period

I have attempted to cover all the important foot-care topics relevant to the general public in this book. However, I realized after talking to many of my patients and medical colleagues that there were still questions that needed answering, but they did not fall into any specific category in the book. Therefore, I have decided to close by sharing with you some of the concerns of my patients and colleagues that were not fully dealt with in the preceding chapters.

QUESTION: You spoke about new diagnostic devices for measuring the biomechanical forces within the feet to determine whether or not a problem exists, or if orthotic devices are working properly. What are they, and how do they work?

ANSWER: The system to which I was referring is called *electro-dynography*. It measures the biomechanical forces on seven different parts of the foot by means of electrodes that are attached on the underside of the foot and lead to a "walking-pack" attached to the patient. This walking-pack stores the information taken while the patient is walking, and the data can be analyzed by a computer, and then interpreted by a biomechanical expert, usually a podiatrist, after it has been printed out. Proper analysis of the information will enable the expert to determine if abnormal amounts of pressure are being put on a part of a person's foot while in stride. It can also be used to ensure that an orthotic device is doing its job.

I am excited by the electrodynogram not only because I love high tech, but because it can tell me more precisely than the human eye whether or not the patient has a biomechanical fault, and, if so, its exact location and severity. Moreover, the procedure is non-invasive. The foot is not exposed to radiation; neither does it have to be subjected to any surgical instrument. Unfortunately, the electrodynogram cannot yet measure precisely how biomechanical faults of the foot can adversely affect the lower-back joints, the hips, or the knees. But I suspect that diagnostic advances will occur in the next few years. Who knows, we may some day be able to predict with a high degree of accuracy where osteoarthritis may strike or have already begun. Orthopedic experts would love to be able to prevent the progression of osteoarthritis to the point where the only treatment left is surgical.

The electrodynogram is the major development in podiatric diagnostic equipment. Even though it is still in its infancy, and is therefore very expensive to purchase and operate, I suspect that it will eventually be quite affordable, and become a major diagnostic tool.

QUESTION: I have seen a few articles about laser surgery recently, and you mentioned it briefly. Can you tell me more about laser surgery on the feet?

ANSWER: *Laser* stands for *L*ight *A*mplification by *S*timulated *E*mission of *R*adiation. A laser device produces a thin beam of light containing an enormous amount of energy that can be focused to remove tiny abnormal areas of body tissue without disturbing or destroying surrounding tissue. One of its earliest medical uses was in the removal of cataracts on the eyes. As far as foot surgery is concerned, it has been used successfully to remove ingrown toenails, warts, and other growths. It has also been used to unblock clogged sweat glands in the foot.

In ingrown-toenail surgery, the use of the laser beam replaces the application of phenol. The beam vaporizes the nail-growing cells rather than burning them. As a result, the healing time is quicker, because the area has not been as traumatized. In fact, laser surgery vaporizes tissue that has to be destroyed, and leaves the area relatively untouched. The problems with laser-beam surgery are that it is still in its infancy, therefore expensive and not readily available, and it cannot yet cut bone effectively. So any surgery involving bone is still in the future, although I suspect that long before I retire, it will become a common practice.

QUESTION: Do you believe in acupuncture and reflexology?
ANSWER: Let me discuss *acupuncture* first. I have studied acupuncture theory, and although I do not use it myself, I have seen some excellent results in the treatment of certain foot problems, particularly neuromas, that would not respond to conventional therapy. I am still not too sure exactly how acupuncture works, but I am quite willing to accept the fact that it can be valuable in the treatment of chronic foot pain.

Reflexology is somewhat of an "in" form of therapy for whatever ails you. I gather that reflexologists believe that by massaging certain parts of the bottom of the foot, certain organs and other parts of the body are beneficially stimulated. As a result, a person will become healthier and stay that way, and possess an overall feeling of well-being with regular foot massages. I have yet to see any clinical evidence that reflexology does what it claims to do, other than to provide a degree of comfort and relaxation. Perhaps much more sensitive testing will eventually be developed to either prove or disprove the claims of reflexologists. However, I must remain skeptical for the moment, although I certainly do enjoy a relaxing foot massage after a long day's work.

In fact, I suspect that the benefits of reflexology are directly related to relaxation induced by the massaging of the bottom of the foot. And, since a more relaxed individual is often a healthier one, there would seem to be a place in the world of therapy for reflexology. I should point out that the same benefits can probably be derived from a mechanical foot-massager—for example, the rolling-pin variety found in certain health-food stores. Another example would be a vibrating foot-bath. All of these devices act in the same way as reflexology: they increase blood-flow into the foot. The increased oxygen supply to the foot creates a feeling of well-being in the area.

QUESTION: Are hot baths good for the feet?
ANSWER: Whirlpools and similar types of hot baths usually feel great, but they can create difficulties afterwards. During a hot

bath the arteries *vasodilate* (open very wide) and allow greater-than-normal amounts of blood into the feet. But for every action there is a reaction. When you get out of the hot water, there is a dramatic *vasoconstriction* (narrowing) of the arteries. Therefore, there is a greatly diminished flow of blood into the feet. This situation could continue for hours if the person has been in the hot water for about fifteen minutes. As a result, there is a diminished supply of oxygenated blood to the foot. A person in that situation, who already has a circulation problem in the lower limbs, will be prone to a number of disorders, as you read in Chapter Eleven. Not only are hot baths potentially unhealthy for the foot, but so are hot-water bottles and heating pads that are applied for long periods of time, such as overnight.

QUESTION: My shoes always wear out on the outside part of the heel. Am I walking incorrectly?

ANSWER: No! It is normal for the heel-strike phase of the gait cycle to occur on the outside part of the heel. Weight is not transferred to the centre part of the foot until almost mid-stance, when the midfoot and the forefoot touch the ground. As a result, there is normal wear on the outside part of the shoe heel—at least for about eighty-five per cent of the population. However, when the weight of the body remains on the outside part of the foot through almost the entire walking cycle, and then switches to the big-toe side of the forefoot, pronation abnormalities occur, and shoe wearing patterns may change. But shoe wear in itself can be misleading; it will not always indicate a weight-distribution problem on the foot.

QUESTION: I was fitted for orthotics and they did not help. I am a runner who does up to thirty miles per week and suffers from chondromalacia (runner's knee), despite having tried most of the running-shoes on the market, exercise programs to strengthen my quad muscles, and inserts in my shoes. My orthotics are two years old. My knee problems are six years old. Why didn't the orthotics do what they were supposed to do?

ANSWER: Orthotics are like antibiotics and anti-inflammatory drugs. Not everybody reacts the same way to the same treatment.

Unfortunately, orthotics do not help everybody, and we have no way of knowing who the unlucky persons will be until they have been tried. Even with the most modern diagnostic equipment for examining the lower limbs, it is not always possible to determine precisely how much a biomechanical foot fault is affecting the knee, if at all. At the sports-medicine clinic where I am the consulting podiatrist, we have been able to determine with ninety-per-cent accuracy when a knee problem is being caused by a biomechanical foot abnormality. Most of these cases respond well with orthotic devices; but I have seen situations where a 10-degree pronation was diagnosed along with a knee problem, and the use of an orthotic actually exacerbated the knee condition. It is unfortunate that you have been one of the unlucky ones. I suggest that further examination of your knee, lower leg, and foot be carried out to determine if some pre-existing condition or intangible factor may have been overlooked.

QUESTION: I get the impression that all biomechanical faults are hereditary. Is that true?

ANSWER: Without a doubt, the selection of parents with foot problems is a major factor—in fact, the most important one. However, there are other causes. The two most common are poor positioning in the womb before you were born, which caused the lower limb(s) to develop improperly, and trauma—that is, an injury of some sort, like dropping a frozen twenty-five-pound turkey on your foot when taking it out of the freezer. The other causes are basically neuromuscular, and are too infrequent to be discussed in detail in this book.

QUESTION: I have been told that I pronate. Will I automatically get a corn or a bunion if I don't do something to correct it?

ANSWER: Pronation describes a mechanical function of the foot. When the pronation is abnormal, the body tries to compensate by itself, as it does with most physical abnormalities. Sometimes the body succeeds, at other times it does not. I have seen people with 9-degree pronation and no side effects, and others with only 3-degree pronation but with corns, bunions, and calluses. The rule of thumb is that about eighty per cent of those who pronate significantly will develop a foot problem eventually. Contributing factors may be the amount of their activity, their style of shoe, or the way their lower leg compensates for a foot fault. We learned in Chapters Fourteen and Fifteen how biomechanical faults are accentuated by physical activities. So my advice to anyone who pronates abnormally and is reasonably active is to have the abnormality treated. The odds are not in your favor that you will be able to avoid uncomfortable foot problems if you neglect it.

QUESTION: I am a sixty-five-year-old diabetic with hammer toes that are causing me severe discomfort. I have been advised to live with the discomfort, because surgery would be risky for me. Is that true?

ANSWER: Diabetics are not necessarily precluded from elective foot surgery, providing that the diabetes is well under control. Theoretically, diabetics are predisposed to impaired circulation in the feet, but this is not always the case. I recently saw in my office a seventy-seven-year-old man who is a controlled diabetic and who has excellent circulation in his feet. There are sophisticated methods to measure blood-flow to a given area; if circulation to the toes is found to be adequate in these tests, there is no reason why a diabetic cannot be operated on for hammer toes, if he or she cannot find relief wearing shoes that have deep toe-boxes. Of course, extra precautions must be taken during and after the operation to ensure that the diabetes is under control at all times.

QUESTION: I am a middle-aged woman in apparently good health. However, for the past few years my feet (and my hands) get very cold and numb at times. My family doctor tells me not to worry about it. Is he right, or do I have some serious circulatory problems he is not diagnosing or telling me about?

ANSWER: Many of my female patients complain of cold feet, even if the circulation in their lower extremities is perfectly normal. I have discussed this problem with specialists in peripheral-vascular surgery, and in internal medicine, and we concluded that the complaint may be due to the fact that the blood vessels carrying oxygenated blood to the foot run deeper in women than in men. Therefore, the skin on a woman's foot is actually a few degrees cooler than that on a man's foot. In this case, cold feet have nothing to do with poor circulation.

However, there is one condition called *Raynaud's syndrome* that affects primarily women, and occurs in cool or cold weather. For some unknown reason, the cold creates a very strong reaction in the blood vessels feeding the fingers and toes. This causes the vessels to go into spasms, which can be very painful, and somewhat serious if the proper precautions are not taken, because of lack of blood-flow to the areas. Victims may also complain that their fingers go pale or blue very quickly when the syndrome affects them in cold weather. Usually the condition is not that serious; if it is, it is called *Raynaud's disease*, and requires immediate attention.

There are some medications that can control the Raynaud's syndrome, but they are not normally required. The best way of preventing episodes of the disorder is to keep your extremities as warm as possible in cool or cold temperatures. If you are concerned about the possibility of having the syndrome, see a doctor for an examination.

QUESTION: You mention exercises for the lower leg, but not for the foot. And you have not discussed the possibility of doing exercises for the foot to prevent abnormal biomechanics. Is it not possible to train the foot to walk properly, so that orthotics will not be necessary to correct a biomechanical fault? I am afraid that if I start wearing orthotics now, I will be stuck with them forever, like an addiction.

ANSWER: First, the overwhelming cause of biomechanical faults is an abnormal position of a bone in the lower limbs, although soft-tissue damage can contribute to the problem when abnormal pronation or supination forces muscles, ligaments, and tendons to overstretch to compensate for a fault. Therefore, there is nothing a person can do to train the feet to walk normally if a biomechanical fault exists; I have yet to see a case where a fault was corrected by an exercise program. My medical colleagues—physiotherapists and orthopedists—agree with me on this point. If you want to *strengthen* the muscles in the lower leg and foot, I suggest that all you really need is a good, brisk daily walk. There is no need to stretch soft-tissue masses in the foot; they are not all that pliable anyway.

Yes, you may become "addicted" to orthotic devices in your shoes. But, consider them as you would contact lenses or eyeglasses. Usually, if you need them, the benefits far outweigh the drawbacks. I believe strongly that we are just in the infancy of understanding the biomechanics of the lower limbs, and that even if orthotic devices today do not always solve a biomechanical problem of the lower limbs, they will no doubt reach a level of sophistication in the future that will mean they can successfully control almost all cases of faulty biomechanics.

QUESTION: You keep talking about shoes. What about socks? Are there certain types of socks or stockings that I should be wearing, or that I should avoid?

ANSWER: I believe in wearing natural-fiber socks—such as cotton or wool—because they absorb perspiration better and protect the foot from the shoe much more than synthetic-material socks. However, as I mentioned in Chapter Eleven, cotton socks are not recommended for people prone to frostbite or immersion foot (chilblain). Women who always wear nylons have little protection from shoe irritation, and from irritation caused by perspiration that is not absorbed. I have one other major concern regarding socks and stockings, and that is size. If you wear a pair of socks that is too short—or even if you pull a pair of socks up too high—you can curl the toes of the foot and enhance the possibilities of developing a hammer toe or mallet toe.

QUESTION: How can I best *prevent* the development of a serious or chronic foot problem?

ANSWER: I have six basic rules I would like to see followed:

1. Learn to recognize the signs of an underlying foot problem, so that it can be nipped in the bud.
2. Wear proper footwear.
3. Practice proper foot hygiene.
4. Do not run or exercise through an injury.
5. Make sure that if you have a foot problem, the diagnosis and treatment are based on the cause of the disorder, and not on

the pain or discomfort itself. Podiatrists, or other foot specialists, are best trained to deal properly with such disorders.

6.   Remember that your feet are the most important method of transportation you have. Don't neglect them!

Index

abnormal pronation, 33-7, 262;
   Achilles tendonitis, 123; aerobics,
   236; bunions, 46-7; calluses, 98;
   hockey, 244; in children, 190;
   metatarsal-head pain, 77-8;
   plantar fasciitis, 119, 120; pregnancy, 170; shin splints, 224-5;
   tarsal-tunnel syndrome, 223;
   tendonitis, 216
abnormal supination, 37
accessory ossicles, 19
Achilles tendonitis, 114, 121ff.;
   aerobics, 237; basketball, 241;
   racquet sports, 238-9; runners,
   219-20; stretching exercises, 125
acid-plaster dressings, 108
acid products: athlete's foot, 135;
   corns, 66; cutting nails, 160;
   warts, 108
acupuncture, 260
adolescent girls: knee pain, 195-6;
   shoes, 202
aerobics, 206, 235-7; shin splints,
   224, 256-7; shoes, 254, 255
airplane flights, 173
alcohol, 173
alcoholic neuropathy, 174
allergic reactions, 139, 144
amyotrophic lateral sclerosis, 169
anhidrosis, 145-6

ankle: ankle-joint synovitis, 223;
   bone, 18, 112; fractured fifth
   metatarsal bone, 94; inversion
   sprain, 238; joint, 20-1; sprained,
   220-3, 241; swollen, 26; turned
   inwards, 94; twisted, 24
anterior-compartment syndrome,
   226-7
antibiotic cream: callused heel, 103
antibiotic therapy: ingrown toenails,
   150
anti-fungal cream, 135-6, 160
anti-fungal pill, 136, 155-6
anti-inflammatory drugs: Achilles
   tendonitis, 125; bunions, 48-9;
   fractured sesamoids, 213; gout,
   167; metatarsal-head pain, 79;
   neuromas, 214; osteoarthritis,
   231; plantar fasciitis, 118;
   tendonitis, 216-17; turf toe, 243
anti-perspirant, 144-5
arch, 18; child's development, 187,
   188; claw foot, 62; fallen, 39;
   high, 39, 116; low, 39; remedial,
   194; support, 44, 131
arteries, 25, 260-1
arteriosclerosis, 25
arthritis, 41-3; fear of, 5, 9; gonococcal, 168-9; gouty, 167; psoriatic, 143; rheumatoid, 167-8. *See*